Dialectical Behavior

Workbook for KIDS:

Introduction

1. **What is Dialectical Behavioral Therapy?**
2. **What is the Goal of DBT?**
3. **Dialectical Behavioral Therapy with Children**
4. **Action Planning and Tasks**
5. **Roles and Responsibilities in Group Sessions**
6. **The Mindfulness Skills**
7. **Interpersonal Effectiveness**
8. **Distress Tolerance Skills**
9. **Emotional Regulation Skills**

Introduction

Over the past decade, Dialectical Behavioral Therapy has become one of the most effective treatments for borderline personality disorder

(BPD) and is particularly effective in treating kids. The effectiveness of Dialectical Behavioral Therapy with adolescents led to many clinicians and researchers exploring whether working with children and families could also be a useful way to help youth. This workbook will focus on how to use DBT skills with your child or adolescent. In doing so, you need to recognize that most of the information found in the literature and on the internet relates to how Dialectical Behavioral Therapy can be used to treat borderline personality disorder. The steps and skills of DBT are identical, whether applied to borderline personality disorder or any difficult life challenge. The difference is when and how those skills should be used.

To work with children effectively, it is important that the kids know their role in therapy, that they learn they are responsible for themselves (even though they feel hopeless), and that they learn exactly what a task involves (it is important for them to have a clear understanding of what needs to be accomplished).

It is also important for kids to know that feelings are not facts, that their thoughts can be distorted, and that they can change their situation by changing their thoughts and actions. They must learn they do not have to be controlled by their painful emotions (e.g., emotions such as rage or despair). Children need to see that it's okay to make mistakes and it's okay to take risks. Children with difficult lives often choose friends who like to get into trouble or are bully-like; these kids also tend to try out new experiences to "feel alive. "

When you introduce the concepts presented in this workbook to your child or adolescent, it is important to remember that they will have very different reactions depending on their level of mentalization. The child will not be able to make the connection between certain thoughts, feelings, and behaviors. If a child is low functioning regarding mentalization, you may find that she does not want to change her thinking or behavior.

When children understand that they can choose to think and behave differently, they will be more likely to try new ways of thinking about and behaving in the world. The child with a more developed sense of mentalization will be more receptive to "the message." They will understand that their feelings are not facts and that their feelings do not need to control them.

The goal for all children is to learn how to live constructively in their environment. When you tell your child that their thoughts and feelings need not control them, you teach them that they are responsible for their behavior. For a child or teen to be able to do this, they need you (the parent) to stop rescuing them from the consequences of their behavior. Parents must act appropriately when kids behave in intolerable ways by setting limits.

The skills presented in this workbook can be used to teach children self-soothing and calming skills, skills to manage their moods, coping strategies for stressful situations, and how to manage the discomfort of urges and cravings.

You can test children and see whether they can understand the concepts in this workbook. When you explain the concepts to a child in the workbook, asking them how they feel about it can be helpful. You will find some kids who are more agreeable than others. You may find that some kids are unsuitable for DBT because they lack the maturity or mentalization skills to understand what is being taught.

When you do use DBT with children, we want to be sure they know it is okay to try different things and that it's okay to make mistakes. Children need parents who give them the freedom to learn and grow. We want to create a parenting style that is not controlling or authoritarian but rather is authoritative; that is, warm and firm. The goal is to help kids become more autonomous and self-reliant while at the same time respecting and supporting their need for safety and security.

The concepts in this workbook are practical ways of teaching children self-control. For children to do this, they need parents who are consistently there for them, support them even when it's difficult, and doesn't react to their mistakes with anger or frustration. Parents must be willing to learn new ways of relating with their children for DBT to work.

Once we understand that DBT is not a cure, the goal is to enable our children to develop more effective ways of dealing with the difficulties in their lives. To do this, it is important to help them understand that what's bothering them can become an opportunity to learn new skills.

We have to help our children develop the coping skills they need and make it safe for them to live in their environment.

If you feel overwhelmed by how complex DBT is, that's okay. We want you as parents to be there for your child or adolescent. To do that, we need you to make it safe for them to ask for help when they need it.

If you're concerned about how your child will respond to DBT training, you may benefit from understanding where their thinking may be off-track first. If you're worried that your child is too angry and unable to learn self-control, this may indicate that they are not getting enough physical touch and affection. Kids who are allowed to get enough physical touch and affection generally develop more effective ways of dealing with life.

To improve how you facilitate DBT training, we encourage you to keep in mind that it's okay for children to try new things, that it's okay for them to make mistakes (they don't have to be perfect), and it's okay for them not to know what the answers are. We want parents to show up consistently for their child/adolescent by being there unconditionally as a parent.

As parents, we have the opportunity to teach our children how to be strong and resilient. We do this by loving them unconditionally, giving them a sense of safety and security, helping them learn how to calm themselves down when they're upset, sharing their feelings with them, and listening to them (not just the words they say, but how they're saying it), and then helping them learn ways of dealing with what's bothering them. Using DBT Skills allows parents to make a huge difference in their child's life.

When you read this workbook with your child or adolescent, it is helpful to go through it together so you can ask them questions about what they are learning. You may find it helpful to have the child do some exercises before you explain them to them.

1.   1.What is Dialectical Behavioral Therapy?

Dialectical Behavioral Therapy (or DBT) is a type of psychotherapy originally designed to treat adults with chronic suicidal thoughts or those with a borderline personality disorder. Dialectical Behavioral Therapy is effective in treating children and adolescents with a variety of behavioral problems:

1. Anxiety

Anxiety is a common disorder that is seen in many children with behavioral disorders and can make it seem hard for them to focus and pay attention in school. When anxiety gets severe enough, it may cause children to misbehave out of pain and confusion at not knowing what else to do. Children with anxiety disorders may also struggle to make and keep friends.

Anxiety is caused by a reaction to an event and often results in extreme behavior as a way to cope. Some of the behaviors children may engage in to relieve their anxiety include:

- Hyperactivity. Children with behavioral disorders may become hyperactive to stay active and feel less anxious. They may also do things their friends find annoying, such as running around all day, bouncing off the walls, or restlessly tucking and folding their arms.

- Compulsive behaviors. When children struggle with anxiety due to poor childhood relationships or abuse, they may engage in compulsive behaviors such as overeating, cutting themselves, overeating, or even hoarding inappropriate material (such as drawing images of weapons).

- Self-harm. Children with behavioral disorders may engage in self-harming behaviors such as: pulling out their hair, hitting themselves, punching, or biting themselves.

Anxiety disorders are the number one reason for medical visits and hospitalization for children. Parents often notice the following:

- Extreme fear

- Trouble sleeping

- Difficulty concentrating and focusing

- Erratic and violent behavior

- Trouble controlling emotions (feelings of anger)

Many children with behavioral disorders report feeling much happier without the constant negative thought patterns that may lead to self-harm, compulsive or hyperactive behaviors, or an inability to sleep. Some children report feeling "nervous" due to overstimulation, familiarity with their environment, or a response to their stresses. Other children may exhibit hyperactivity due to poor childhood relationships, or lack coping skills to deal with Outside influences such as drowning and fire are common triggers for anxiety in children. Hormones, diet, and genetics can also play a role in the onset of anxiety symptoms.

Like adults, many children report having early memories of anxiety or an inability to control emotions. Because family dynamics and other events often influence childhood memories, recovery is often seen in the form of allowing the child to acknowledge their feelings and develop new skills when necessary. The goal is to help children express their feelings without acting on them (or sharing them with others). The therapist can help the child develop new ways of acting as well as recognize behavioral triggers that may lead to feelings of anxiety. For example, a child afraid of the dark may benefit from learning how light therapy can be used instead. Triggers may be learned as a new coping skill, like using a visual timer to help count down from ten seconds before bedtime.

DBT is not a cure but a significant step forward in helping children cope with anxiety. It teaches children how to think about feelings and use alternative methods of coping if they are overwhelmed by their emotions. The goal is not to change the child's behavior but to help them understand it so they can move on to healthier coping skills. It may take time, but these skills can be learned and have a lasting impact on a person's ability to cope.

2. PTSD

Children who experience trauma or abuse may develop Post-Traumatic Stress Disorder (PTSD) or other types of anxiety disorders. Kids who have been sexually abused may develop PTSD and exhibit some of the following symptoms:

- Nightmares

- Flashbacks

- Trouble sleeping

- Feeling lots of anger, sadness, and confusion

DBT teaches children methods for dealing with their emotions without feeling overwhelmed. The goal of treatment is to help the child learn how to express these feelings in a safe environment. The child will learn to identify triggers that may result in negative emotional reactions and practice new coping skills when those triggers are present.

3. ADHD

Children with ADHD may display various symptoms that make paying attention and controlling their emotions difficult. These children often have trouble with schoolwork and may feel like they are different from those around them:

- Difficulty paying attention in class

- Inability to stay seated and still

- Lack of focus

- Trouble listening to instructions

- Difficulty remembering what they are doing or where they are supposed to be going. This often results in the child being late due to forgetfulness or running out of places quickly.

Children with ADHD often feel like something "wrong" with them, causing them to criticize themselves and others around them. Children who feel like there is a problem with ADHD may also exhibit the following symptoms:

- Night terrors

- Excessive fear of bodily harm, especially during sleep.

Teenagers are often misdiagnosed with ADHD when they have Adjustment Disorder or other types of anxiety disorders. These children often have trouble coping with stress and may resort to "acting out." Some teens experience severe depression or suicidal ideations when their lives are filled with conflict and stress. Others feel like they just don't fit in anywhere and act out by engaging in self-harm behaviors such as cutting, burning, or punching themselves. Sometimes the teen self-medicates by abusing alcohol or drugs to help cope with the issues in their lives. Anxiety disorders can be debilitating to a teenager, but the good news is that developing new coping skills can help these teens move forward.

Psychotherapy often works well for teenagers who are struggling with anxiety disorders. CBT helps teenagers learn how to recognize their feelings and use coping skills to deal with them in a safe environment. For example, when a teen feels like they just don't fit in, they may benefit from learning how to write out their feelings to express themselves and overcome those feelings by coming up with solutions on how to improve self-esteem or find one's place in life. Getting rid of negative emotions is the goal of treatment, but it may take time and patience before those new skills pay off. DBT helps teenagers manage their emotions, but the real goal is to move beyond the negativity and learn how to deal more healthily.

4. OCD

Obsessive Compulsive Disorder (OCD) often affects children in a way that makes them feel like their thoughts control what they do and say. They may:

- Avoid certain places or situations because it makes them feel uneasy.

- Feel like they must perform certain tasks or rituals to prevent negative outcomes. For example, a child who feels compelled to wash his hands excessively may avoid using public restrooms so he won't come into contact with germs or dirt.

- Feel like they are responsible for the actions of others. When a child with OCD feels responsible for something bad that happens to someone else, they may engage in behaviors such as excessive washing or counting to eliminate the bad thoughts.

- Think that something bad will happen if they don't perform certain rituals or follow certain routines. Children with OCD often feel like negative things will happen if they don't complete their tasks (checking the stove twice before bed or ensuring all the lights are off before leaving a room).

The goal of treating OCD is to help children replace their obsessive behaviors with more positive and productive ones. Mood-boosting medications and antidepressants may be used to help children cope with their stress and anxiety.

5. Panic disorders

Panic disorder is often characterized by episodes of strong feelings of terror and irrational or "uncontrollable" fears. Children may have:

- Panic attacks where they feel like they are dying or experiencing extreme anxiety. The child may feel dizzy, lightheaded, and disoriented by these attacks.

- Feelings that they are being followed while in public places such as shopping malls, restaurants, or schools. They may feel like something is "wrong" with them or that the world is closing in around them, causing them to panic and begin to hyperventilate. They may begin to sweat, shake or tremble and exhibit other anxiety symptoms such as trouble breathing, chest pain, or choking sensations.

Children with Panic Disorder often feel like they are different from other children and may blame themselves when something bad happens. They may also feel like they are not good enough or that others won't like them if they reveal their true self to others. Because these children experience panic attacks almost every day and find it difficult to cope with their emotions, treating the anxiety is essential to helping them improve their self-esteem and coping skills.

6. Depression

Depression affects the emotional and mental health of children. The symptoms of major depression can fall into four categories including:

- Depressed mood (feeling sad or empty)

- Reduced energy and enthusiasm for activities

- Reduced interest in previously enjoyed activities or hobbies

- Significant change in weight

Depression often begins as a child's normal mood ebbs. When the child starts to feel pretty good, they may notice that their "fun" side is gone. In addition, the child may begin avoiding situations where they might otherwise enjoy themselves. For example, a child who normally enjoys playing outside with his friends may spend more time in their room instead of sleeping and eating.

It is important to note that when children feel like they can't get positive feelings, they may not be experiencing depression and need to be evaluated by a doctor. Often children display signs of depression long before they stop getting out of bed or interacting with others in the school. While it is not always easy to change how a teenager feels about themselves or feel like there is nothing wrong with them, these children must receive treatment for the disorder as soon as possible.

Treating an Anxiety Disorder

Tips for treating anxiety in children:

- Develop new coping skills. Teach your child how to use coping skills to calm themselves down when uncomfortable. These might include breathing exercises, positive affirmations, meditation, or visualizing peaceful scenes. Techniques like yoga are also beneficial.

- Learn about triggers. Some children with panic attacks may benefit from knowing: What sets off their panic attacks or what factors in their environment may make them uneasy (such as certain sounds). Knowing what sets an anxiety attack off can help the child avoid these triggers and calm themselves down when they know they are coming "down."

- Be mindful of safety issues. Children with behavioral disorders can get injured when they act impulsively due to feelings of anxiety. Avoid leaving your child alone in situations where they may get hurt, such as crossing the street or playing sports.

- Talk to your child. Using "I messages" may help build self-awareness and communicate feelings: "I can see that you are feeling anxious." Children who are afraid of their panic attacks may benefit from calming themselves down if they recognize that the attacks are bodily responses instead of dangerous events (for example, "It's okay, this is just a panic attack.")

- Never ignore symptoms. If your child feels they have had enough, let them have time out. If they continue to feel anxious, try to redirect their attention. You must take them to the emergency department if they continue acting out.

- Support your child. Children with behavioral disorders may not have the same peer support as adults. Take time to build a strong bond with your child before therapy begins. This bond helps children feel comfortable and safe during sessions.

- Foster a sense of self. Empower your child by building skills that help them learn about themselves and develop empathy for others. Find ways for them to express their emotions without acting on them or sharing them with others.

- Make sure there are no underlying medical or genetic issues. If your child has a history of trauma, anxiety attacks, or behavioral disorders, consult with a doctor and consider getting a genetic test.

As you can see, there are a lot of disorders that can affect children and teenagers. Anxiety disorders have become a serious problem for children and teenagers, making schools and families the place where they need to feel safe and safe from their worst fears. Finding effective treatments may take time as an individual develops new coping skills over time and through participating in therapy sessions. DBT therapy has shown promising results in these situations and is often the most effective treatment of anxiety disorders in children. DBT works by teaching the client new skills and helping them to identify patterns of unhealthy or destructive thinking and behaviors that lead to problems like mood disorders or self-harm. Clients learn new skills and strategies that help them manage their emotions through distress tolerance, interpersonal effectiveness, mindfulness, and behavioral regulation. These are crucial areas as they are essential for self-harm and mood stabilization. As with many other disorders that affect children, anxiety disorders can seriously affect the child's emotional and social well-being. Sadly, they are often overlooked or simply not taken very seriously. Parents should be aware of these signs and symptoms in their children and seek help if they suspect they are suffering from an anxiety disorder.

The treatment requires a lot of commitment from the therapist and the client. It requires hard work, consistency in practice, and dedication from both parties to see positive results. DBT does not have any quick fixes or magic answers. It takes time for the client to learn new ways of thinking about life events, react differently in those situations and respond differently when they begin feeling distressed.

DBT has the following parts:

1) Individual psychotherapy: The therapist works with clients to change their thoughts, emotions, and behaviors. This is done by analyzing the client's patterns of thoughts and actions as well as listening to the clients describe their problems and behaviors. The therapist helps them understand their emotions, how they came about, and how they impact the client's life.

2) Group therapy: Therapists will work with clients individually and in a group-based format to help them cope with their problems. Clients may also participate in group therapy only if they request it from their therapists or choose to do so on their initiative.

3) Telephone coaching: This group session allows clients to practice their skills as they learn them. This can be done either once or several times per week, depending on the client's needs and treatment progress. It allows clients to ask therapists questions, address situations that may be difficult to address in therapy, and provide feedback on their progress.

4) Skills training manual: DBT is based on specific skills and strategies for emotional regulation and behavior change. The manual provides detailed information about each skill, its purpose, how it works, and how it should be used. Therapists coach clients through their use of these skills so they remain consistent in applying them when needed.

5) Education sessions for family members: DBT therapists will provide family members with education about the disorder and its treatment. This helps them to know how to support their loved ones in treatment,

which is especially important for children with BPD. Family members are also taught how to apply skills at home and determine when they should seek professional help if they need it.

6) Relapse prevention: Relapse prevention is an important part of DBT as it prepares clients to recognize symptoms of relapse and makes them "more resilient" to these situations. A client's therapist may identify places where they experience high levels of distress, areas in their life prone to self-injurious behaviors, or relationships where the client is likely to act out. Therapists help clients to recognize these triggers and learn how to address them appropriately.

7) Crisis Intervention: In cases where a client displays extreme distress or suicidal behavior, therapists work with the client and family members to provide support while contacting emergency services if necessary. Clients are not discharged from the program until they feel stable and ready to return to normal routines.

Unlike some other therapies, DBT is based on the theory that clients' problems are not fixed and must be approached from the start of accepting the problem. Since DBT was first developed for people with Borderline Personality Disorder, it can be more challenging for children to participate in DBT because either of these conditions may be present in children.

Even though a child is not diagnosed with BPD, if they are displaying behaviors similar to those found in a person with BPD, this would make them eligible for DBT treatment. DBT was designed for adults, so there are some challenges to making the treatment specifically tailored for a young person's needs.

DBT therapists work to personalize the therapy to fit each child by using the information gathered in a functional analysis, which is an assessment to determine why there is an ongoing problem. Suppose a child is not diagnosed with BPD but has similar behaviors interfering with their functioning. In that case, they may still be eligible to participate in DBT even if it is not the most effective treatment. DBT recognizes that everyone is different; therefore, each person's treatment plan will vary based on their needs.

Dialectical Behavioral Therapy Skills and Strategies

The main skills taught in DBT are emotion regulation, distress tolerance, and interpersonal effectiveness.

Another skill is called "The Life Space." This skill is used to help the person examine their life from three perspectives: past, present, and future. The past life space focuses on understanding all the experiences that have led a person to where they are today, and the present life space looks at what a person needs right now to get through their difficulties. The future life space looks at how people can change themselves tomorrow to continue on track with their goals and values.

These techniques can benefit any child struggling with interacting with their peers, staying on task, and following through on tasks they have already started. These skills can also help a child deal with their anxiety and the resulting depression. It will allow the child to think about what they are doing more clearly, understand that they can solve their problem, and learn how to help themselves.

Some of the strategies used to teach these skills include:

1. Hypervigilance: This is when a person is very aware of their environment and everything around them. This can help a child focus better on what's happening in school or at home, but it can make it difficult for them to relax and enjoy activities like playing video games or watching television.

2. Emotion Regulation: Learning to recognize their emotions and their triggers, the child can then learn how to manage those emotions, so they do not interfere with their ability to function. The child will learn techniques to cope with those emotions, such as deep breathing, practicing mindfulness, going for a walk, or doing some reading.

3. Distress Tolerance: Sometimes the things that are going on in their lives are a challenge to their mental health, and instead of allowing themselves to get overwhelmed and give up, they can now use these skills to learn how to take care of themselves at the moment and then try harder in the future.

4. Interpersonal Effectiveness: This is a way for them to communicate better with others, so they can be more successful at asking for what they want directly or compromise with others when there is a conflict.

5. The Life Space: Using this skill will help them see their experiences from different perspectives, which will help them make sense of those experiences and figure out what steps need to be taken next.

DBT can be a very effective method for helping to manage a child's problems with mood, personality, and behaviors that cause distress in their life. Some children with BPD do not require the full DBT system but may need to use some skills and strategies. This is also true for children who do not have BPD but display similar behaviors and can benefit from DBT.

1.　　　　2.What is the Goal of DBT?

What does DBT focus on? Dialectical Behavior Therapy aims to help children and adolescents who struggle with emotional trauma and behaviors resulting from their psychological pain. DBT strives to teach adaptive skills that decrease impulsivity and increase coping skills by teaching children how to regulate overwhelming emotions more constructively.

DBT strives to help children develop emotional regulation skills to live more rich and more meaningful lives. DBT recognizes that each person is different, and emphasizes the individual strengths of each child, how the child views their world and how it affects their behavior. DBT also acknowledges that problems do not occur in a vacuum and focuses on understanding how our thoughts and behaviors affect the world around us.

DBT is a type of therapy that helps people manage their emotions. DBT can help kids who have difficulty expressing themselves or have difficulty managing frustration, anger, sadness, or other intense emotions. It teaches kids different tools to help them manage difficult situations and to be happy with themselves. These tools help them learn to understand their negative feelings and how to control them.

DBT teaches children to understand and accept their emotions rather than try to change them. It helps them change the way they behave when those emotions come up. This type of therapy is based on the idea that our thoughts and feelings are interconnected. Therefore, to change behavior, it's not enough to change how we think—we must also learn how our thoughts affect our behavior.

One of the biggest challenges for young people is managing their intense emotions. DBT teaches kids to express their feelings and accept the consequences of their actions without expecting things to be different in the future. It also helps them learn how to cope with difficult situations like losing a friendship or teasing others. It teaches them how to relate well with other people and how they can express what they want in a way that doesn't upset them. This lesson will help kids develop healthy relationships while they are still quite young, which can help keep those relationships forever.

DBT teaches people how to tolerate their painful emotions and tolerate the difficult situations that often cause these emotions. It helps them navigate their distress healthily so they can cope with it long-term.

The main goal of DBT is:

1. To teach kids how to change their behaviors. The most important part of changing behaviors is coming up with a list of specific goals you want to accomplish. If you don't know the goals, it's hard to work on them.

2. Teach kids how to accept and like themselves, even when they make mistakes or mess up. Many kids with behavior problems also have things they are uncomfortable admitting or showing to others. They might feel like they are bad or weird. This kind of thinking and feeling, called "shame," can make it hard for them to change their behavior.

3. Helping kids to relax and cope with whatever is going on for them at the moment. When people are stressed out about something, whatever it is doesn't go away, but we often start doing things that make us feel worse instead of better. Sometimes we fight with other people; sometimes, we melt down or shut down and have crying or tantrum episodes. Sometimes we engage in self-destructive behaviors like drugs or cutting. We will have more emotional control and better handle stress when we work on these behaviors.

4. To teach kids new ways of relating to other people. Sometimes the way we interact with other people is not very effective in reaching our own goals. We often push, cajole, demand, or frustrate others into

doing what we want. This makes it hard for them to relate to us; they may do things that make us angry or hurt, leading us to have more intense emotional reactions that push others away even more.

5. To help children have more peace of mind and less stress in their life. By learning to stay calm and focused, they will have fewer emotional reactions that make it hard to get what they want in life. They can learn to pay attention to the most important things and figure out how to make those happen.

Many kids come into therapy because they have trouble with their emotions and relationships with other people. Sometimes they feel like they can't control their behavior or understand themselves very well, especially when upset or angry. They may do things that make other people angry, but they don't know why. They may not know what their personal goals are in life or how to work on achieving those goals. They often feel like someone else is controlling them or making them do things, which makes it hard for them to figure out what they want for themselves or how to get it.

Therapy can help them understand these things and use them to change their life. It can be a safe place to share their feelings, learn new ways of thinking and behaving, and develop healthy ways of coping with life.

The skills learned in therapy can help children feel better about themselves. They will have new tools to handle stress and difficult situations in life and work on making themselves more important to others. They will learn to accept themselves for who they are now, even if it's not the perfect person in the world (because no one is). They will understand why other people act the way they do and see things from their point of view. They can assert their feelings and wishes without fear of what other people will think about them. They might have more friends and better relationships with family. They will feel more in control of their lives, which means they will be happier.

The challenge of understanding and effectively responding to a child's mental health problems are serious. Few people in our society have been formally educated on child/adolescent mental health issues. Many teachers have little or no training in recognizing when difficulties are beyond their scope of practice. The lack of proper understanding and training in diagnosing and treating mental health issues can lead to the under-diagnosis of children and adolescents.

It is very hard sometimes to understand our child's behavior as parents. We must not blame ourselves or become frustrated with our children. We must take the time to learn more about these problems and how they might be affecting our child's life. Suppose you are unsure of what is happening when your child becomes upset or angry. In that case, it might be a good idea to seek the advice of an experienced professional who can help you understand what you can do to help better manage your child's emotions and behavior.

Ways Dialectal Behavior Therapy Can Help Parents

1. Learn how to manage their own emotions. Some parents don't know how to prepare themselves for raising kids. They might be very sensitive, easily overwhelmed, and get stressed out by the smallest things. DBT teaches them new tools for managing their emotions to function better as parents and care for their kids more effectively.

2. Learn to control interactions with other adults and children better. Often parents are very reactive since they don't have much control over their children's behavior or emotions. Children can be manipulative and demanding when upset or angry, making life very hard on adults unprepared to handle those moments. They can also be quite clueless about how to handle these situations. DBT helps them change their behaviors so they can get what they want and make other people feel better about themselves. They will find ways to resolve difficult situations with kids that are healthy for them and ensure that the kids behave in ways that don't upset or hurt others.

3. Learn new coping strategies for stressful events; instead of asking "why," parents will be taught how to understand and cope with their children's emotions and behavior when upset or angry. Sometimes things cause anger, sadness, jealousy, etc., but not everyone reacts similarly to a stressful event (or even a different reaction from another person). Parents will understand how to deal with these events more effectively to help their children better.

4. Help the family work together to work out issues with each other and resolve conflict. DBT helps families learn new ways of

communicating and working together that are healthy for everyone. This can help kids feel safe dealing with difficult situations. It also helps parents feel better about communicating with each other in ways that don't upset or frustrate each other, which is good for everyone.

5. Help them have more peace of mind, so they have fewer emotional reactions and are not as prone to stress-related diseases like diabetes, obesity, heart disease, depression, etc., at young ages. DBT helps parents understand what stresses them out and how to avoid those things that can cause problems for their kids. This helps them feel better about themselves and prevents many health problems like diabetes, obesity, heart disease, depression, substance abuse, and more at young ages.

6. Help them better understand the problem behaviors of their kids. Many families aren't aware that their children have problem behaviors like anger, aggression, lying, and drug/alcohol abuse. Sometimes parents don't know what to do about the problem behaviors. DBT helps parents understand these behaviors better so they can work on helping their kids change these things and learn healthier ways of interacting with other people.

7. Help them overcome fears, especially some of the very common fears like death, abandonment, or being alone. Often parents are afraid or anxious to go through certain things in life like death, abandonment, and being alone. These are something that most

people experience at times in life, but many people don't want to deal with those feelings.

The therapist's role in the therapeutic process is to help the child clarify what they are thinking and feeling, clearly understand their goals, and work toward achieving them. It can be difficult for a child to communicate with adults because they may not have the words or the cultural knowledge needed to explain how they are feeling. It can also be hard for parents who don't understand what their child needs help with.

When children cannot explain their feelings, they may act out, which might be disruptive or aggressive. Or they might withdraw and isolate themselves, so they don't have to deal with their problems. Either way, these behaviors make it difficult for children to live an enjoyable life with other people and feel good about themselves.

A therapist can help a child navigate these situations by helping them understand what is bothering them and how it's making them feel so they can resolve the conflict healthily. It's difficult to figure out what is wrong sometimes because our feelings can get mixed up with how we feel about ourselves or the people around us. Sometimes we can't determine what we want or how to get it.

A therapist can help a child understand these situations by helping them see how the conflicts they are experiencing impact their life and their ability to reach their goals. This will help them learn how to adjust their behaviors to be more effective in getting what they want.

Children have a lot of feelings inside themselves that can get mixed up and make it hard for them to know what is going on with their emotions. When a child has problems recognizing their feelings, they might start to feel very emotional in certain situations and not know why. Or they might start having emotional outbursts because they can't regulate the emotions inside of them.

A therapist helps children understand how their feelings work to identify better what happens when they are upset or having problems managing their emotions. This will help them to stay calm and think more clearly when dealing with stressful situations.

1.   3.Dialectical Behavioral Therapy with Children

Dialectical Behavioral Therapy with children is similar to other types of talk therapy, but the techniques are usually more specific to children. For example, children in therapy are encouraged to reflect on how they feel instead of just reporting their thoughts and feelings.

Although DBT is effective for children, it can take time. For DBT to be effective, there needs to be close rapport between the therapist and the client. The therapist must see which parts of DBT fit a child's problems best. There are many reasons a person might choose DBT over other forms of therapy with children. One reason is that DBT is a "whole person approach." Dialectical Behavioral Therapy works with a client's strengths and can be tailored to fit a child's personality and needs. Another reason DBT might be helpful is that DBT is geared towards behavior problems, like aggression or emotional regulation problems. Dialectical Behavior Therapy incorporates medications and other therapeutic techniques but does not overuse them. They are there to support the client, not replace them.

Children who undergo Dialectical Behavioral Therapy often benefit greatly from it. Many children who receive therapy through schools have fewer discipline problems and better social skills than before they started therapy. In addition, children who do not get support from their families due to abuse or neglect usually have fewer behavioral problems after DBT.

If you suspect your child needs a therapeutic approach for emotional problems, advocate for your child to receive Dialectical Behavior Therapy. The steps are simple:

Step 1: Find a therapist who uses DBT for children. Ask them to give a "backward history" of how they would treat your child's behavior problems and how long it would take to get a therapeutic effect.

Step 2:   Study the therapist's approach. If it seems appropriate, ask the therapist to explain the basic ideas behind DBT, such as "validating" feelings and total acceptance of life circumstances.

Step 3:   If you like what you see, arrange an appointment with your child and ask them what they think of the therapist's approach. Also, have them ask some questions if they have any. It's important that your child is interested in therapy, or it may not be an effective treatment.

Step 4:   If everyone seems to have the same understanding of DBT and the therapist is willing to use this approach with your family, ask the therapist for a cognitive behavioral therapy plan and schedule of reviews.

Step 5:   Continue seeing the therapist until you are satisfied with their work. If the therapy isn't working for your child, consider trying another therapist or approach.

Doing what you feel is right for your child would be best. If you want them to get better and they aren't improving while in therapy, consider having another conversation with the therapist. You can be the one to say that you think therapy isn't working.

A good therapist will be open to that conversation and do their best to try different techniques so that your child can get the help they need.

DBT can be a powerful tool to help children with emotional problems. If you think your child might benefit from this therapy, remember that it's okay to advocate for your child to receive the right treatment. It might just make a huge difference. Remember, you are your child's biggest advocate. Say something if you feel they aren't getting better or the therapy negatively affects them. You know your child better than anyone else, and you must stay involved in their care if something doesn't feel right to you.

How does DBT work?

To understand how DBT works, it's important to know what it is trying to do.

In general, Dialectical Behavioral Therapy focuses on helping a person either:

• Express feelings in healthier ways • Change behaviors that harm themselves or others • Improve their ability to tolerate distress

For example, your child might have a lot of anger towards other people. This might be expressed through screaming at them or hurting them. If your child can learn new ways to express their emotions without violence, they will feel better, and so will the people around them. DBT tries to achieve this type of change with most of its clients.

Another example of a problem that DBT tries to help with is disruptive behavior, such as temper tantrums. Children with destructive behaviors like this often cause problems at home and school. If your child can learn new skills to help them stay calm, they will be able to improve their relationships with others and do better in school.

DBT is based on the idea that all people, even children, can change themselves for the better. This means that thinking about how you feel or what you need is not a bad thing. It means that we are in control of our lives, and we can make changes for the better if we choose to do so.

The goal of DBT is not to remove all emotions and feelings but to help a child understand what they are feeling and express it in ways that don't hurt anyone.

How does Dialectical Behavior Therapy work with children?

There are many ways that Dialectical Behavior Therapy can be helpful for children. Because children are growing and changing, DBT needs to be flexible and adapt to different situations.

When talking with your child's therapist, one important thing to remember is that they are there to help your child. Therapists understand that sometimes you need to vent or that you might not like how your child acts. They will listen and allow you to say what you need, but they won't agree or disagree with it unless it has something to do with their work with your child.

DBT therapists use a combination of children's emotion regulation skills and behavioral skills. This means they will help your child learn how to cope with their feelings and express them healthily. They also teach your child how to stop behaviors that are bad for them or harmful to others, like having temper tantrums or being disruptive at school.

How does Dialectical Behavior Therapy work with teenagers?

In most cases, DBT may not be a parent's best choice when trying to help a teenager with emotional problems. While DBT can be helpful for many children, it is not as effective for teens because it doesn't focus on helping teens change their behaviors as it does for children.

DBT can be a good fit for children ages 7-12 because it is geared towards helping them learn new coping and coping skills that are appropriate for children. For teens, the focus of DBT changes from learning new skills to focusing on helping the teen accept their emotions and thoughts without judging themselves or their behaviors. This is a hard task for teenagers, who are still developing their sense of self.

If you are considering DBT as an option for your child, remember that it isn't always the best choice and should always be combined with other approaches like Cognitive Behavioral Therapy or Family Therapy. There are many types of therapy, and no one type is better than all the others.

Many parents feel frustrated when they see their child isn't doing better after starting therapy. Sometimes it's easy to get frustrated because we know how much our children struggle, and we want to see them get better quickly.

It's important to remember that every person is different, and what works for one person might not work for another. It can take time for any therapy to start working, and sometimes it takes a lot of different approaches before you find the one that can help your child the most.

Remember that there are people who are here to help your child, and you are your child's best advocate. If you keep that in mind, and it can take time for therapy to work, you can work through any frustrations or worries. How do you know what will work for your child?

You might want to try a few different approaches before you decide on one. Remember, each person is different; what works for one person doesn't always work for someone else. Different approaches can be effective in helping your child learn new skills to help them cope and change the behaviors that are hurting them or other people.

It's important to discuss your child's progress with their therapist as often as possible and make sure they feel comfortable talking to you about what they see in your child. It's important to keep the lines of communication open, so both of you know what is working and what isn't.

When talking to your child's therapist, make sure you understand the goals they would like to help your child achieve. It's also a good idea to discuss your thoughts about what might be causing the changes in your child that you're seeing. If you understand what is going on with your child and try a few different things before deciding on one, it will be easier for everyone involved.

Common complaint parents have about therapy is that their children don't seem to be getting better. This is an important issue because any therapy has to be evaluated regularly and adjusted if it doesn't seem to be working. While it can be frustrating to see your child struggle, it's important not to give up until you have tried every option.

Never feel guilty if you decide that a certain type of therapy isn't working for your child. It isn't always easy to find the right fit, so keep an open mind and try many different things until you find the right one for your child.

DBT is an effective form of therapy for many different kinds of problems. If you are interested in learning more, many different types of support groups can offer help and advice.

DBT isn't as effective with older teens because it is geared toward helping them learn new coping skills, and teenagers haven't mastered the skill of coping skills. They must learn to accept their thoughts, feelings, and behaviors without judging themselves first. They also need to learn new skills for social and academic situations to be better equipped to deal with the inevitable challenges of being a teenager.

If your child is in a position where they have a lot of support from their family and the school, they might not need therapy as much as it's commonly thought. If you think your child has a lot of emotional struggles, talk to them about therapy at their next well visit.

You might even want to try starting with just one type of therapy to see if it works before you commit yourself to finding an all-inclusive therapy package for your child.

When you start therapy, it can be very important to work on your child's self-esteem and encourage them to have a good attitude about their struggles. A great way to do this is for you and your child's therapist to develop a series of affirmations that your child can repeat.

For example, every time your child has a good day at school, encourage them to be proud of themselves and tell them how much you appreciate their hard work. Please help them to understand that it is okay to stumble and sometimes fall because we are all human, but the important thing is to try our best.

It's important to remember that if your child feels like they have support from family and friends, they will probably do better than they think they will. If they believe they have help from those who love and care about them, it makes everything much easier.

If you or your child's therapist notice that things aren't going well or somebody is getting frustrated with a therapy approach, switch gears. It can be frustrating when they keep trying the same thing, and nothing seems to help or change.

As long as therapists work with the right approach, it would be best if you didn't give up on therapy immediately. When we see our children struggle, we often want them to improve immediately, but it's important to remember that therapy takes time. You need to keep trying because it doesn't work every time.

It's important to keep in mind that DBT can't work overnight. It takes time and effort to learn new skills and change old behaviors. It's also important to stick with treatment or change plans because they might take some time to help. If things don't seem to be improving, you or your therapist might want to make a change.

But don't give up! When done correctly, DBT can be very effective in helping people like you manage intense feelings and deal with the problems that cause those times. If it doesn't help at first, keep trying different types of therapy until you find a good fit for your child that will work for their needs. Finding a therapist with experience working with children is important because certain factors differ from adults in therapy, such as age and development.

What problems can DBT treat?

DBT hasn't been shown to cure mental health problems, but it does help many teens manage their behavior, feelings, and other symptoms to lead better lives. It can also help with anxiety, depression, eating disorders, and many other common problems.

DBT Tips For Managing OCD, Selective Mutism, and Repetitive Behaviors

Dialectical Behavioral Therapy with children with depression and anxiety disorders is an evidence-based treatment that can be very effective for those with difficulties with emotions, behavior, and other problems. If you are a parent or caregiver of a child struggling with mental health issues, it's important to work together with their therapist so they can learn new skills to manage their emotional problems.

The following tips will help you work with your therapist and deal with your child's problems as a parent.

DBT Tips For Managing OCD, Selective Mutism, and Repetitive Behaviors

1. Don't let your child give up when they feel overwhelmed by emotions. If they feel stressed and upset, encourage them to find different ways of dealing with their difficult thoughts and behavior to get them through their problem.

2. Help them see that not everyone reacts similarly to any situation. Try explaining that one person might feel sad, angry, or anxious about a situation while another will act out in another way. Children need to understand that every person is different, and sometimes we don't know why we react one way when other people react differently.

3. Acknowledge that not everyone feels the same emotions all the time. Children with anxiety or mood disorders tend to feel sad, angry, or upset for long periods. If your child feels like they always feel bad, it might be helpful for them to understand that we don't always feel the same way all the time. Sometimes we feel good, and sometimes we feel bad; it's normal to experience both feelings.

4. Don't let your child use their emotions as an excuse for acting out in inappropriate ways. While it's important to help children manage their emotions and learn new skills, they shouldn't use those emotions as an excuse when they are inappropriate in situations. They must develop appropriate ways to express themselves.

5. Help them see that emotions aren't always easy to control, and it's okay to feel upset sometimes. Everybody has times when they are overwhelmed by emotion, and it's okay for them to feel that way. As long as your child doesn't hurt others and does not stay in a bad mood for too long, it's okay for them to be upset.

Children struggling with intense feelings and behaviors might find this therapy helpful if they have a therapist or clinician with experience working with children like them. It's also important to remember that

DBT doesn't just help people feel better by focusing on one feeling or problem. Instead, it helps them learn how to handle problems and feel better about themselves. You must help your child understand the DBT process and how it can help them solve their problems. While it may take a lot of hard work, your child can learn new skills and ways to manage intense emotions.

1.   4.Action Planning and Tasks

Action planning and tasks are often designed to teach children two types of skills: how to behave and stay calm. Together, these skills will help guide your child through a highly emotional situation in a healthy way. The good news is that children can learn these skills quickly and easily

Why Do We Need to Teach Action Planning and Tasks?

Children have a lot of things to deal with in their lives, especially between the ages of 8–12. The world is unpredictable, with many challenges and obstacles, but children learn to handle it much sooner than adults ever expected. Adults can now be considered late bloomers compared to children because children are exposed at a much younger age than ever.

Children have very complicated life and have a lot of emotional experiences. As a result, they can act in ways we would not expect from someone their age. In addition, children are very sensitive and emotional creatures who are overwhelmed by so much at such a young age. In some cases, children are so emotionally and mentally exhausted they are unable to function in day-to-day activities.

Teaching action planning and task skills gives children and adolescents the ability to act with actual consideration of consequences. Studies show that children who use action planning and task skills are less likely to act out negatively when feeling frustrated, nervous, or angry.

Teaching action planning and tasks for kids will help them stay relaxed, happy, and healthy but also help them handle their emotions more appropriately during high-stress situations. Dialectical Behavior Therapy (DBT) tells us that the earlier we begin teaching children how to manage their emotions, the better off they will be in the long run. The sooner we start teaching these skills to our children, the more they will be able to handle all other aspects of their lives and these emotions.

According to DBT, children need to learn to become more effective problem solvers. They need to learn how to calm themselves. This will be especially important during times of stress or crisis in their lives.

DBT tells us that kids don't start developing self-help skills, such as the ability to calm down and stay calm, until they are at least eight years old. Babies cannot yet control their own emotions and choose what actions they take when emotional states occur. DBT also teaches us that this does not happen in the brain but is a learned behavior from parents, siblings, teachers, and caregivers from early childhood to adolescence.

DBT suggests that it is vital for parents and teachers to teach these skills to children at a young age. The earlier children learn to react calmly during a crisis or highly stressful situation, the less likely that child is to develop depression or other mental illnesses later in life. These are skills your child needs now and will need in the future. Just like adults need these skills to function effectively in their lives, so do children! The sooner we can teach these skills, the better.

For action planning and tasks to be effective for children, caretakers must establish clear boundaries around what behaviors are appropriate and what should be off-limits. For example, it's important to instruct, "I want you to speak calmly at all times," and "It's not okay for you to push anyone or yell at them until they calm down." Remembering these rules will make it easier for your child when they need them the most.

The following examples illustrate how action planning and tasks can be implemented to help children deal with difficult emotions. Remember that your child's situation will determine which skills you will teach them.

Directions – this type of task is just what it sounds like: saying out loud to your child a series of directions (e.g., "turn up the television, sit at the table, take all your toys outside, put your coat back on"). Tasks like this one can be done in a manner that takes care of the immediate need for direction (which tends to happen when children are in an emotional state), or they can also be modified so that they teach more useful skills (e.g., "go get a drink of water, then come back and brush your teeth").

Name – there are times when children need to be reminded of the names for things (e.g., "I want you to use a different language when we're at home so we can both understand what you're saying"). There are also times when it's useful for children to have their name called out, followed by an action that the child needs to take (e.g., "look at my face, then look at your ball and put it down." Reminders like these can also be combined with some activity to teach your child

Evaluate – there are times when children need to be told what to notice about their behaviors (e.g., "notice that you're crying, you are so angry right now, notice the way your body feels"). Similarly, it's often useful to coach children by asking them questions like "why do you think you're _____ (sad/mad/angry) right now?" or "what do you think would happen if you _____?". Directions like these can be combined with other types of tasks (e.g., "I want you to notice that you're crying, I want you to notice how your body feels, and I want you to notice the way your body feels while you cry); they can also be combined with other skills (e.g., "I want you to use a different language when we're at home so we can both understand what you're saying"); or they can take the form of a statement (e.g., "you feel so angry right now, if we don't calm down, it's going to harm us both."

Defend – this type of task is used to teach children how and when to defend themselves against something that's going on immediately. For example, a child might be given a ball and told, "I want you to throw the ball at me so I can catch it; what does throwing it at someone mean? If someone is threatening or pushing you, that's the situation where you need to throw your ball at them". Children will learn how and when to defend themselves by practicing this kind of activity over and over. They will also learn how to behave while defending themselves (e.g., they shouldn't push back or hurt anyone else).

Reflect – This task teaches children how and when to reflect on what happened. As with defense, there are times when children will be given objects (e.g., dolls, action figures) and asked to name various body parts while reflecting on what happened. In addition to this type of activity, it can also be productive to coach children by asking them questions like "how do you feel right now?"; "what did you do when _____ happened?"; or "what would you like me to do with my body when _____ happens?"

Review – This task teaches children how and when to review their actions. For example, your child might be asked to imagine that they're in a time machine and can see themselves doing something. Then, they will be asked to tell you what they did, and then they'll be asked to repeat this information calmly. Tasks like this one can be combined with other types of activities (e.g., "I want you to use a different language when we're at home so we can both understand what you're saying"; "I want you to notice that you're crying, I want you to notice the way your body feels, and I want you to notice the way your body feels while you cry").

Empathy – this type of task is used in Dialectical Behavioral Therapy for children to teach them how and when to respond empathetically. For example, your child might be asked to imagine that they're in a time machine and can see themselves doing something. Next, they will be asked to tell you calmly what it must feel like for them. Tasks like this one can be combined with other types of activities

Teach – this type of task is used to teach children how and when to teach someone else. For example, your child might be asked to imagine that they're in a time machine and can see themselves doing something. They will then be asked, "what do you want to do with your body when you do that?". Tasks like this can be combined with other activities (e.g., "you look very tense, what do you want to do with your body when you look that way?).

Calm – this task teaches children how and when to calm themselves (e.g., using deep breathing). It also can be useful as a tool for learning theme words (e.g., "how do I act when I am calm? What should I be doing with my face? What should I be doing with my body?"). Activities like these can also be combined with other types of Dialectical Behavioral Therapy tasks

Set limits – this type of task is used in Dialectical Behavioral Therapy for children to learn how and when to set limits for themselves and others. For example, your child might be asked to imagine that they're in a time machine and can see themselves doing something. Next, they will be asked, "should I have said that?" or "should I have done that?". Tasks like this one can be combined with other types of activities

Create a relationship with oneself – this type of task is used in Dialectical Behavioral Therapy for children to teach them how and when to create healthy relationships with themselves (e.g., how and why they should be angry or sad). For example, your child might be asked to imagine that they're in a time machine and can see themselves doing something. Next, they will be asked, "how do I feel about what I did?" or "why did I feel that way?"

Recognize – this type of task is used in Dialectical Behavioral Therapy for children to teach them how and when to notice different situations. For example, your child might be asked to imagine that they're in a time machine and can see themselves doing something. Next, they will be asked, "what are the consequences going to be of what I did?" or "why do these things happen at all?". Tasks like these can also be combined with other activities (e.g., "what do I do when _____ happens?").

Create a relationship – this type of task is used in Dialectical Behavioral Therapy for children to teach them how and when to create healthy relationships with others. For example, your child might be asked to imagine that they're in a time machine and can see themselves doing something. Next, they will be asked, "how can I become friends with _____?" Tasks like this can also be combined with other activities (e.g., "I want you to get along with me more than anyone else, how can we do that?").

Identify the triggers – this type of task is used in Dialectical Behavioral Therapy for children to teach them how and when it's helpful for them to identify the sources of their negative emotions. For example, your child might be asked to imagine that they're in a time machine and can see themselves doing something. Next, they will be asked, "how did I feel when _____ happened?" or "what emotions do _____ make me feel?". Tasks like these can also be combined with other activities (e.g., "if you look sad, what are all your feelings in the situation?").

Wants – this type of task is used in Dialectical Behavioral Therapy for children to teach them how and when to want healthy things. For example, your child might be asked to imagine that they're in a time machine and can see themselves doing something. Next, they will be asked, "what would it be like if I wanted ____?" or "what consequences will there be if _____ happens?". Tasks like this one can also be combined with other types of activities

Your child may feel that you are too strict and controlling when setting up available tasks. They may not like doing them and will want to push back by arguing with you. In these situations, it's important not to get upset but instead remain calm and firm with your child. Stay the course and show your child that they have no choice in the matter. Eventually, they will learn that compliance is better than resistance.

Healing from trauma or past mistakes can take a long time if someone is not teaching your child healthy coping skills. Being calm when upset or angry is just as important as learning how to act appropriately in a given situation.

The idea is that if your child can keep themselves and others in a calm state of mind, they will find that they are capable of doing things without struggling.

Tips for Setting Up Your Dialectical Behavioral Therapy Tasks

You'll need to set up your tasks as quickly as possible, so you don't lose momentum by using them too much. Eventually, you will want to create more and more complex tasks for your child to learn from.

Step 1: Start with something simple. Your child will have difficulty (or at least need) becoming accustomed to the task before adding more pieces. So, start with something they can do right now instead of saying, "When do you want to start doing that?" or "When are we going to do this?"

Step 2: Give them a choice on how they want to receive feedback on good behavior. Allow your child some time and space when they have completed their tasks for them to reflect on and talk about what they have done well or not so well. This will help them to make the correct adjustments for next time.

Step 3: Give your child a choice on how they want to receive negative feedback. This can also be combined with other tasks (e.g., "I want you to _____, what behavior do I need to use for you to stay calm?"). Always give your child clear and concrete instructions about how you want them to behave in the future (i.e., "I want you to start telling the truth, so when do I need to know that a lie has been told?").

Step 4: Be alert and firm, but not angry or forceful. Set a clear timeframe for the behavior you want your child to learn and when (e.g., "I will allow you to be angry or upset for ten minutes, then I will ask you to say three nice things about yourself").

Step 5: Be prepared with a positive reinforcement system. This system includes having your child complete certain tasks (e.g., I like how you finished your homework, I notice how hard you are trying here). It also includes giving them some of the things they desire (e.g., I love how healthy and peaceful those two are, they look so happy together).

Step 6: Use positive reinforcement systems again and again. This will help strengthen the behavior you want them to learn.

Step 7: Modify the tasks for your child's skill level. If your child is a beginner, try setting up some simple tasks to help them get started on their way to mastering something. If they're advanced, start with more complex tasks that will teach them how to do things better or faster. You can also move back and forth between these two types of tasks while they are progressing through learning these new skills.

What are the Benefits of Action Planning and Tasks?

As your child learns to use action planning and tasks, they will have a more structured experience with emotions. These skills will help your child learn to manage their emotions constructively and productively. At school, your child will get positive feedback from friends and teachers. Your child will be more effective in solving problems of many different kinds, regardless of size. In the future, your child may even decide that they want to pursue a degree in therapy. Your child will have more practice with new skills and life experiences than most children at this age. This experience will help them stay calm at home, school, work, and other situations for the rest of their life. Action planning and tasks make everything more manageable. The result is that these skills will build your child's self-esteem and confidence. By learning these skills, your child will feel better about themselves and how they handle emotions.

As time goes on, your child's exercise of these skills will become more natural. Your child will have fewer problems at school, and they may find their grades improving. Your child may have fewer problems getting along with family members and friends. Your child may even lose any fears of other people and situations. As time goes on, your child may enjoy opportunities for socialization and improvement.

You will find that your work as a parent gets much easier as well. You will have fewer problems with how your child acts or reacts, so you will spend less energy in arguments, fights, and other situations that create conflict in the home. Kids who can do action planning and tasks are more confident about what they do at school, home, sports, art projects, etc. Children who do action planning and tasks are likely to be more willing to risk emotional hurt more constructively. Children with these skills are less likely to end up in the justice system. Action planning and tasks make it easier for your child to understand why they feel afraid or angry, which will help them learn more about emotions and develop self-esteem. Action planning and tasks give children this experience at home with you, where they can practice their new skills. This will help them see how they can manage their emotions, so they don't use them in destructive ways at school or other places.

Action planning and tasks are essential for kids to develop their language and cognitive development. They must have these skills to build a healthy language acquisition process. It's also essential for them to develop fluency and fluent speech in the future. Action planning and tasks are critical aspects of social socialization and survival, coping with group dynamics, etc. It's a tool that will help them cope with the stress of everyday life.

Undoubtedly, children with action planning and tasks are more successful than other children. They can survive better in society and are more successful overall at home, work, or school (depending on their age).

1.   5.Roles and Responsibilities in Group Sessions

Group sessions in Dialectical Behavioral Therapy for children are structured so that every participant can talk, listen, and share. It is a principle of DBT that everyone in the group has an equal voice. Young children sometimes forget their turn to talk or share how they feel and need reminders from the therapist or peers to participate. Due to their age, young children do not always recognize the importance of sharing their feelings or problems. They may also be afraid or unsure how to express what is happening inside them. Strategies can be taught to help children healthily express themselves during group sessions. The therapist or other peers prioritize maintaining eye contact and engaging young children in ways that they find entertaining, enjoyable, or comfortable. This creates an environment where young children feel safe and want to participate in further discussions.

The therapist also teaches young children how to listen to other group members. This may include teaching them how to take turns and share with others in the group or by having them share what they are thinking, feeling, or want to do next. Young children may often get distracted by their thoughts and talk about the wrong thing.

They may think too much about what is happening inside themselves and not enough about their feelings and problems. The therapist will try their best to teach strategies that can be used when things get messy or when young children have trouble following directions, as well as techniques that can prevent young children from getting too anxious when there are multiple thoughts, feelings, and ideas being shared at once.

Sometimes parents or adults may feel that the children are not participating appropriately. This is usually due to a lack of understanding of what is expected. For example, adults may feel that a child should be talking more. However, suppose you remember that every person in the group has an equal voice, and every person has an opportunity to talk. In that case, it may be easier to understand why they seem reticent. Parents/adults need to respect the skills and experience of the therapist when it comes to how a group session is run. Remember that most therapists have worked with children for many years before becoming DBT therapists and have experience with many different methods of working with children in group sessions.

Each child's role is usually first decided by rank, with the person with the highest rank speaking first. The person with the lowest rank may have other responsibilities, such as handing out materials, cleaning up craft materials, taking notes during discussions, or even counting votes during decisions about group rules and procedures.

Two co-facilitators lead groups with different backgrounds and skills. The co-facilitators take turns leading the group and managing the schedule. Generally, the co-facilitators do 90% of the talking during a session, encouraging everyone else to speak. Participants need to talk to identify their thoughts, feelings, and beliefs about what is happening. This helps them better understand themselves and others at home, school, and work.

At the start of a group, children are asked if they have any questions about the group. It is important to reassure them that they will be allowed to ask more questions as this will be useful for them later in the session with their therapist. Parents are generally allowed to ask questions on behalf of their child at this time as well.

Younger children are often unaware that they have to wait their turn but should know that not everyone has the same number of turns. It may be helpful for an adult to remind children that it is very important for everyone to have a turn and that no one should feel bad if they do not get a chance to talk.

When children are allowed to ask questions, it is important to give them a prompt before their turn so that they can take their time and think about the question. It may be helpful for adults to wait with the child until they have finished asking the question, although this is usually not necessary for younger children. It is very important for the child asking the question not to rush through their words to make progress on a transition. Asking questions allows children to learn how to set up future group conversations.

Adults must provide the therapist with a list of questions that the child easily understands. For example, if the question is about what to do when someone gets angry, adults may ask their child how angry s/he gets and what s/he does or says after a fight. Young children often ask questions like "when am I going home?" that could be better asked at home. It is also helpful for parents or adults to offer group members work on their own that young children can be given at home, so they do not feel pressured into staying in a group situation.

What happens when children behave badly in the group?

Children are not punished or rewarded for speaking in therapy. However, they may sometimes notice that the therapist will want to speak to their parents/adults in private or ask other children or adults to talk with them privately if they have used words like "hate" or "kill" towards someone else. If this happens, you need to let your child know that you spoke with the therapist about their feelings and how worried you were about what they said. It is also important for you to let your child know that it is okay if they want a break from DBT if they are scared or upset by what happened.

Children may find that they have put what they have been thinking into words and that this is scary. Some children may use words like "kill," "shoot," or "stab" when they are angry or upset. This is not intentional, but it can be hard for them to notice because these are how people talk when angry.

Because DBT focuses on not using these words, children may sometimes feel foolish for using such words. They may also be scared if someone with a weapon pulls on them or tells them something like this when they are upset.

If a child is having trouble with self-injury, it can be helpful to have the therapist meet with parents/adults and explain things they can understand. This can help parents/adults to be more supportive of their child, and parents/adults who have been through this may also feel more confident in helping their child.

Most children can use DBT in the long term. The therapist will monitor the children's progress and make adjustments during treatment if it is necessary for their safety or that of others. Children should never be encouraged to use revenge or hate towards people who hurt them or cause them harm.

Individual Roles and Responsibilities

Children may take on different roles depending on what is going on in the group (for example, during a discussion about being nice to each other). The younger and more inexperienced the group members, the more likely a chart will be used to explain different roles and responsibilities.

Children must know their feelings and can be able to share what they are feeling at any time during the group session. The therapist may create a scene using toys or draw one. To talk about feelings, the therapist can then use emojis to demonstrate how they feel when they are happy, sad, angry, or scared.

If children feel uncomfortable, explaining the situation to them may be a good idea, so they do not feel that they are being a nuisance. Once the group is in session, children are asked if they want to speak and share their thoughts and feelings. They may also want to speak in small groups without being called on by others. Once this has been established, the group can discuss difficult topics such as bullying or understanding why someone is being mean.

If you have a time limit for the session, you should talk with your therapist about how long it will take for all children to have speaking time during each session. Adults may feel frustrated if the therapy is not working fast enough or their child's behavior is not improving. It may be helpful to remember that everyone heals at a different pace. Each child has a different background, and it may take longer to learn new skills than anticipated. Sometimes children and adults do not respond to treatment as you expect, which does not mean that Dialectical Behavioral Therapy is ineffective. Everyone responds differently, so it's best to be open-minded about what works for your child and family.

It is very important that parents/adults are fully supportive of the group process and actively encourage their child to participate. It may also be helpful to get feedback from the therapist on how they think they might be able to improve a particular aspect of the treatment, such as their role in the group or when more practice is needed.

If your child is not having an active role in the group, it can be useful to remind them that everyone has an equal voice. This may make them feel better about not being called on so much. Children can feel intimidated by other children who appear older or have more experience with DBT than they do. Asking the other children to take turns can help everyone feel more comfortable. It may also be useful to ask children how they learned something new, what helps them to stop and think before they act, and how they manage their emotions when someone says something mean.

Tears, tantrums, or disruptive behavior during a group session are normal. When children do this, they need support from their therapist and peers to calm down. Everyone should be reminded that there are no bad feelings and that expressing them at any time during the group session is acceptable. It may be helpful for parents/adults who are upset by these outbursts to consider whether it is related to something upsetting or stressful in their lives.

Actions taken by children when they leave a group session are important to the success of the treatment. It can be helpful for parents/adults to remind their children that the therapist helps them learn new skills and that it is okay to use these skills at home.

The therapist reminds children when it is time for a break and helps them check on how much talking has been done. When children have finished speaking, they may take turns with other children in small groups discussing different topics, such as being nice to each other.

Generally, children leave the group session feeling listened to, heard, and understood. They often feel better about the situation, are more willing to talk to others at home and in school, and better understand themselves and their relationships with others. They also better understand what is happening in the group and have found that they are not alone with their feelings.

The therapist may want to follow up with children at home following a group session if you think it would be helpful for them to do so. Parents/adults may also be invited back into the group as guest speakers or observers if they feel this would be helpful for their child.

If you are asked if you would like your child to participate again next week, you must make sure that they know how well they did in the session before letting them know whether this is something that your family will continue.

The pace of your child's responses can vary daily, so you mustn't feel pressured into deciding on the treatment if you are unsure what is going on for your child.

It can be useful for parents/adults to record how well their child does in the group over several weeks or months. This may help to give parents/adults some idea of how DBT works for their children and how long it will take them to learn new skills and change their behavior.

When children have been with the group for some time, they are sometimes asked if they would like to become a co-therapist. They are asked to help the other children and adults in the group to feel more comfortable and willing to share their feelings.

Remember that doing Dialectical Behavioral Therapy is not an easy task, but it can certainly be worth it. Just like learning any new skill, you need to put in the time, practice, and effort before you will see results. If your child struggles to get the most out of DBT or is having difficulty participating in a group session, it may be useful for you to talk about these issues with your therapist.

The therapist will try to maintain an appropriate tone of voice and respect in the group. Even though some children may be difficult to work with and might not be interested in following directions, the therapist will respect their voices and questions. The therapist will also make sure to use a manner that elicits positive responses from children when speaking with them. Suppose a child tells the therapist that they are worried about something and are scared or worried. In that case, the therapist considers this as when a child shares information about their day or wants to talk about story books or what they have eaten for lunch.

Children work at their own pace in DBT. This may be a very fast pace for some children, while it can be slow and steady for others. Some children may be helped by having a therapist always there to offer encouragement and support and answer their questions. Other children may like being called on in groups, whereas others will not respond until they have had a chance to think about what they have heard or seen.

If you decide it is time for your child to no longer be part of the group, the therapist will work with you to find another child interested in joining them in the next session. The therapist will encourage you to be sure that this child is ready for DBT but also ready to share their feelings.

Children with more than one therapist often like having different ones they can switch between. This helps them adjust and feel more comfortable with the therapist they are working with at any one time.

Many parents and children find that joining a DBT self-help group is a great way to connect with others dealing with similar difficulties, build new friendships, and learn new skills for managing their emotions in healthy ways. It can also provide parents and children with a safe place to share how they are doing with one another. A self-help group may be the best fit for some families, as it allows family members to practice and learn new skills on their own time.

A therapist may also recommend that the young child complete their behavioral chart at home. These are often used for homework assignments for children to practice using DBT skills. Parents are advised to use the charts with their child at home and praise them each time s/he makes progress. The therapist should explain to the child that it is their job to manage themselves and should not be used as a punishment by the parent/adult.

The therapist may also recommend that an adult use a behavioral chart with their child. This will allow parents and young children to manage their emotions healthy while learning new skills when apart.

During this time of development, parents may experience some initial resistance to the idea of letting a child have a positive emotional experience without their presence or that seeing a therapist is not healthy. Parents need to remember that they are modeling their behavior to their children and that it is often easier to give in to situations if others around them do so. This can happen with your child or another child in your care, even if s/he comes from another family or school. Many parents will find themselves reluctant to express anger directly at the therapist if they know their child's therapist may have the same anger issues and will thus be more likely to communicate with therapists of similar backgrounds.

As a general rule of thumb, avoiding taking your child out of the group is best if you are frustrated with them during the session. Your child should stay in the group and have the therapist work with them one-on-one, or it might even be helpful to remind yourself that they are not therapy and everyone will recover differently. However, suppose your child cannot manage their emotional functioning. In that case, it is important to consider this when making decisions about whether your child should remain in a specific setting or be referred for individual therapy.

As with any mental illness, parents need to speak with their children's therapist about how the child is feeling and how their progress is going. It is often helpful for therapists to set up a time each week to call the parent(s) of patients in a DBT group to check in with them consistently. This helps the parent feel more included in their young child's treatment and allows them to address any concerns.

Many feelings and behaviors associated with BPD can also be found in children, from intense fears to overwhelming anger. It is often helpful for parents to recognize these behaviors for what they are, watch out for them, and work on how they might express their emotions.

The roles and responsibilities in group sessions are essential. Suppose a child or adolescent is unwilling to take responsibility for their behaviors and emotional functioning. In that case, they will likely be unwilling to do the work in therapy too. The therapist will also be able to step in when a child does not want to participate, but that would be extremely rare. The therapist will almost always encourage the child to ask questions, support their feelings and help them manage any difficult feelings and behaviors so that s/he can access the skills needed to deal with them in healthy ways. All these things help children manage their emotions in healthy ways and feel better so they can learn new skills.

The role of a therapist is to help young clients identify and change negative behaviors, increase self-awareness, build coping strategies and improve overall emotional health. The therapist will be there for the child and their family for as long as necessary or until the child can make the changes that s/he needs to meet the family's goals. By making such changes, it will be possible for them to make greater strides in meeting the goals that have been set for them by their family and their therapists.

1.   6.The Mindfulness Skills

Mindfulness is a way of paying attention to life in the present moment without judgment. It can be as simple as focusing your attention on the flow of your breath. When you are mindful, you are fully aware of everything happening around you. When you concentrate on your mind and body, you will notice what's happening inside of it and how it feels.

When children practice mindfulness exercises, they notice the thoughts coming and going in their minds. Instead of getting involved with those thoughts' negative or positive nature, children will see them for what they are: just words or images in their heads. When the thoughts come into children's minds, they can observe them instead of sticking to them or trying to stop them. If a child notices that he is being selfish and doesn't pay attention to what others want, he can wait until later to make amends.

Mindfulness skills help you be present now by paying attention to your thoughts, feelings, and surroundings. The skills teach you to observe your thoughts, feelings, and reality without getting attached to them. They help you focus on the present instead of worrying about the past or what might happen in the future. For children, taking care of their thoughts and feelings is particularly important. This helps them to handle stressful situations in their life that they may not have control over, such as illness, divorce, etc. Mindfulness skills can also help children with ADD and ADHD. These children are too focused on the present, which results in problems paying attention and controlling their behavior.

Mindfulness has been proven to be an effective way of treating anxiety disorders in both adults and children. It helps individuals stay calm even during stressful situations. If children learn to be mindful at a young age, they can carry this trait throughout their lives.

Mindfulness is more than just an emotional process, but it is also a self-regulation process as well. When you are mindful, you are more able to control your actions, emotions, and thoughts compared to when you are not mindful. Self-control is an essential skill that helps a child to do the right thing and not give in to their urges, even when they are tempted to do it.

Children can practice different forms of mindfulness: observing themselves, their reactions to a situation, and their body sensations. Children can alternate between these three activities depending on what they need. Some teachers will have children practice mindful breathing or keep a journal of their thoughts to write out any worrisome thoughts or feelings as soon as they occur. This helps them learn self-regulation and use those skills throughout their life. Another way for children to practice mindfulness is through meditation. A way that is simple for a child to participate in.

Mindfulness skills are helpful for children because they can help them to become more aware of their thoughts and feelings as they are happening. This helps them to slow down and think about what is happening rather than just acting on their thoughts immediately. It helps children to understand the difference between what is true for them and what is not true in their life. Children can practice mindfulness exercises when they have a stressful situation or if their mind gets away from them because of their current activities.

The Mindfulness Skills in Dialectical Behavioral Therapy

Dialectical behavior therapy (DBT) is a type of cognitive behavioral therapy that focuses on the specific problems that affect someone with a borderline personality disorder. A person with this disorder can get caught up in certain negative thoughts and feelings or even actions, regardless of the consequences. DBT focuses on helping people identify their emotions to learn how to understand them better and accept them instead of getting overly involved with them. It also helps people to understand why they are experiencing these emotions and be able to change their behavior as a result.

The mindfulness skills used in DBT are divided into the following categories:

1. Observing

Observations are an important part of mindfulness activities because they teach children to observe themselves without judgment or opinion. Children can practice seeing their thoughts and feelings as they are happening, so they do not get overly involved or try to avoid them. This helps children to have an objective view of themselves and their experiences.

Observing is a skill where children learn how to watch what is going on in their minds. They practice being aware of the thoughts in their head and the things they are feeling at a given moment. They also practice being aware of what they see, hear, touch, taste, or smell in their environment. When children learn to observe what is happening around them, it helps them process information better and responds to situations appropriately.

2. Describing

When children learn how to describe what is occurring in their minds, it helps them to learn more about themselves and what they are feeling. It also helps them to be able to observe without judgment. When children can describe their thoughts and feelings, they can put some distance between themselves and their emotions. This allows the child to deal with the emotions in a better way rather than letting them control them.

Describing is telling someone else what you think and feel at a given moment without judgment or opinion. It can help children to watch their automatic thoughts instead of getting caught up in those thoughts or trying to push away painful thoughts altogether.

3. Participating

When children can participate in an activity, it helps them to move away from their thoughts and feelings and instead pay attention to their surroundings. This allows children to learn how to put some distance between themselves and the emotions that occur when they are getting involved with their thoughts.

Participating teaches a child how to acknowledge what is happening around her without judgment or opinion on the situation. They can observe without being bothered by the negative emotions around them.

4. Nonjudging

Nonjudging is a skill that helps children recognize how their thoughts and feelings are impacting them without judgment or opinion. This helps them to be more aware of their emotions and thoughts as they are happening and become more aware of the things that make them who they are. It allows a child to understand their behaviors better; by doing so, they better understand the situation around them, increasing their ability to respond appropriately.

Nonjudging teaches children how not to have judgments on themselves or others around them. When a child does this, they can limit the number of negative emotions they experience by not getting overly involved with those emotions.

5. Self-validating

Self-validating helps children understand and accept reality without any judgment or opinion on reality itself. When children practice self-validating, they can better understand why they feel the way they are and how to identify and accept those emotions.

Self-validating is a skill that helps children to understand that their thoughts, feelings, actions, beliefs, choices, and behavior do not have to reflect what others want them to be. Self-validating teaches children how to validate themselves without judgment or opinion on others around them or the situations they are in. Self-validation is learning how to accept themselves and where they are in life while being aware of the things that make them who they are.

6. Empathy

Empathy is a skill that helps children understand how they can better relate to others. It helps them understand how they should act around others and their feelings. It teaches children how to acknowledge others' feelings and the importance of being sensitive to those feelings. Learning empathy allows children to recognize when someone needs help, even when it may be hard for them to do so. They can take control of their actions and not react due to the actions of others around them.

Empathy is learning how to relate to others healthily so that you can act accordingly. It helps children learn to keep everyone's feelings in mind and not react immediately in situations involving other people. When a child practice empathy, they can take control over their emotions and know how to act accordingly so they can deal with the situation appropriately.

Mindfulness skills build focus, personal management, and self-awareness. Mindfulness is a great way for children to build concentration and attention span, which can be beneficial in the classroom setting. It fosters a sense of cooperation with others by fostering empathetic skills in children at a young age. It teaches them how to empathize with others and let their emotions go while helping them practice being aware of their feelings and thoughts.

These skills help children realize what they can do when they feel negative emotions such as anger or sadness so that those strong feelings do not control them. When children practice these skills, they can build awareness of their feelings and thoughts to cope with them properly. When children learn to let go of their negative feelings and emotions, they can calm themselves down to better deal with any problems.

By using mindfulness skills, children learn how to take control of their thoughts and emotions to better deal with the stressful situations around them. These skills help children recognize the importance of early awareness to build a foundation for concentration and attention span. It helps children learn how to cope with stressful situations to prevent them from happening again.

Mindfulness helps build discipline and self-control in children, which is extremely beneficial when learning new tasks or general education. It teaches them how to recognize their stress and emotions so they can properly deal with them. These skills help children learn how to calm themselves down when they are in a stressful situation, or that causes them to feel negative emotions.

When children practice mindfulness skills, it helps them realize what they need to do to better themselves, which builds confidence. It gives children the ability to know what skills are needed to better deal with problems and the reassurance that they can get through whatever issues arise.

Children who practice mindfulness better understand their surroundings because it teaches them how different mindsets affect their actions and behaviors. This can help children recognize their attitudes, thoughts, and emotions and realize what causes them to become more aware of those things. When they practice mindfulness skills, they can take control of their emotions and deal with problems that arise in their lives.

By practicing mindfulness skills, children can better understand other people's feelings and the importance of being empathetic. It helps children internalize those feelings so they know how to act around others or when an unfamiliar situation arises. These skills teach them how to deal with situations so they don't become overly stressed or upset, greatly benefiting children in school and life.

Strategies Used To Teach Your Children Mindfulness Skills

1. Put Mindfulness on the Schedule

Mindfulness skills are something that should be taught at an early age. Children need to learn these skills because they will greatly benefit them. Children need to understand that they can use these things every single day and that it is a valuable skill that can help them deal with stressful situations in their life. By having mindfulness on the schedule, children will see how they can benefit from these skills and how they will affect them in their daily lives.

2. Use Themed Activities

Give your children fun activities for school so when you tell them about mindfulness, it can relate to their life and make learning something more fun. When you use them to teach your child mindfulness skills, they will be able to understand the concept of mindfulness and how it applies to their daily life.

3. Make Mindfulness Part of Their World

Mindfulness is a very important skill that children need to learn, so find different activities for them to do for them to apply mindfulness to their lives. Children need to experience different activities that will make them more mindful of their world. Give your children different activities at home so they don't get bored with learning about mindfulness and can apply it in their daily lives.

4. Start Small

When teaching your children mindfulness, start with an activity that will not overwhelm them. Children tend to get overwhelmed, so give them activities that aren't too difficult for them and will help them learn to be mindful. This will allow them to connect with the concept and apply it to their lives healthily.

5. Be a Role Model

Set an example by practicing mindfulness yourself. Children watch everything their parents do, so they learn better when following your lead. They need to see that you are also being mindful so that they can learn how to apply these skills to their daily lives.

Mindfulness can be used in any aspect of life, from school, home, and even work. Mindfulness skills are thus essential, not just for school but also treating yourself and for many other reasons. Now that you read about the benefits of these skills, you will know how beneficial it is for children to develop their mindfulness skills.

So, what are you waiting for? We can live a much more fulfilling life by cultivating the habit of being mindful in everything we do. Practice these mindfulness skills with your kids and make them aware of their importance in everyday life. It can help them grasp the concept early so they can have a firm understanding as they grow older.

1. 7.Interpersonal Effectiveness

Interpersonal effectiveness is the ability to understand and deal with other people appropriately. Children must be taught how to effectively manage their relationships and interactions with others to develop positive relationships in both childhood and adulthood. This principle can be learned with good coaching. Behavioral and cognitive therapists provide good coaching to help children develop effective interpersonal skills to manage their interactions and relationships in childhood and adulthood.

Interpersonal effectiveness in Dialectical Behavioral Therapy (DBT) is a skill that can be taught verbally and nonverbally. Children can learn effective interpersonal communication skills in DBT with good coaching by behavioral therapy professionals. Children can effectively communicate their needs and preferences when they learn their skills. The children can work with their parents and therapists to develop effective skills of interpersonal effectiveness.

Interpersonal effectiveness is a set of communication strategies taught in DBT that help individuals function effectively with others. Effective interpersonal behavior helps people be self-sufficient and make decisions based on good logic. One of the core skills in interpersonal effectiveness is one's ability to "request" or "say no." It is also important that a person has good coping skills if they are being bullied or demeaned or if they are being asked by a teacher how to accomplish something.

Childhood interpersonal skills can include developing a "friendship contract" with another child. Children need to have the skills to form positive relationships with others and develop friendships. It is a skill that can take time to learn, so parents need to be patient and support their children while learning how to interact with others in healthy, effective ways. A good friendship contract often includes expectations and boundaries that might include no name calling, no stealing or breaking things belonging to other children or agreeing on how much time on an electronic device such as a computer, iPad, or iPod would be appropriate. Once the expectations are set in writing, both parties must follow through on the agreement.

The skills that children learn to manage and interact with other people in childhood and adulthood can be positively impacted by the good coaching of behavioral therapists. Interpersonal effectiveness skills are also important in relationships with professionals such as teachers and other people you are interacting with regularly. The therapist must teach how one goes about talking to these professionals without becoming frustrated or annoyed. It is also important for the patient to know not to become defensive about how others are treating them.

Many people deal with a negative or critical social exchange in their lives. The goal of DBT is to teach skills that will assist persons in managing negative interactions, internally and externally, so they can learn how to tolerate those situations better and improve their quality of life.

The following are specific skills used to achieve interpersonal effectiveness:

1. Proactive communication:

Proactive communication means that the child is aware and can control the interactions they will have with others. It involves being able to use and regulate emotions, as well as clearly defined goals, plans, and intentions. Effective communication means that a child can explain their thoughts to others in detail and maintain their boundaries within the conversation.

2. Problem-Solving:

Children need to be taught how to solve daily problems at school, at home, or playtime. Children who are given a problem and told "solve it yourself" will understand how things work and learn from mistakes made so they can make better decisions next time.

3. Active listening: Active listening involves listening to what others say and responding in a way that shows you understand what they are saying. This skill is important to develop because it teaches children how to problem-solve and how others feel about something.

4. Assertiveness:

Assertiveness is a skill that involves having your own opinions and beliefs without hurting anyone's feelings. Children need to know when it's appropriate to say "no" and stand up for themselves without putting down others or saying hurtful things.

5. Speaking effectively:

Children need to be able to find the right words for the situation and convey their ideas in a way that will get others to understand what they mean. This skill is important because children would have difficulty expressing their thoughts and ideas without it.

6. Managing anger:

Anger is a feeling that everyone has, but it needs to be controlled. Children need to learn and understand why they feel angry and how to resolve their anger healthily. This can be done by listening to music, writing their feelings on paper, or even doing physical exercise.

7. Handling conflict productively:

Conflict is always a reality, but it doesn't have to be a negative experience. Conflict may mean two people don't agree on something, or someone might not feel respected. Whatever the situation, conflict is inevitable, and children need to be able to handle it productively.

8. Handling criticism:

Children who can handle criticism are better at being realistic with themselves and their goals set for the future. They can accept changes and see them as opportunities rather than failures. Suppose a child isn't able to handle criticism well. In that case, they will likely avoid situations that involve it, which can lead to an unhappy future with few opportunities for success.

9. Forgiving and making amends:

Children need to learn how to forgive and make amends when they are wrong. Forgiving others is one of the most important things a child can do because it teaches them that even though mistakes have been made, forgiveness does not diminish the severity of the situation. Children should learn to accept their failures positively without blaming anyone else.

10. Using self-talk effectively:

This skill involves controlling thoughts and feelings so you can effectively converse with yourself or others. It also involves knowing how to listen to your inner voice and what it will say in different situations, so you can make better decisions for yourself or others without ignoring your feelings or thoughts.

These skills help children make good decisions, choices, and judgments in all situations. They give children the ability to make the right decisions in their lives, so they don't make mistakes that affect them negatively. These skills are lifelong and will help children feel fulfilled in their lives.

Interpersonal effectiveness is essential because people will only want to work with others who will make a difference in their lives. People need to be able to make the right decisions based on how well they get along with others, and children must learn these skills as early as possible. This is one of the most important aspects of success in life.

Children need to know that their teachers and parents are there for them and will help them succeed in school. However, children also need to feel good about themselves so that they aren't put down by others and suffer from low self-esteem. This is an important skill so that children can have confidence in themselves that they don't let other people down by being dishonest or showing disrespect towards them.

As people, children need to know how to live up to the noble standards they have set for them, so they can feel successful and accomplish all their goals. There are many different ways in which people can grow through life, but these skills can help children with these matters.

Interpersonal effectiveness is very important because it helps people get along better with others and live better lives. Interpersonal effectiveness involves making decisions based on how well you get along with others, and this will help you deal with problems that others may make for you in life. This skill will help you make good decisions based on how you feel others may be affected by your decisions. If you don't get along with someone, then you won't know how to interact with this person.

This skill is very important because it helps people know how to listen to others and respond in a way that will not offend anyone else. This skill is also important because it teaches children what they should say in different situations so they don't cause problems with teachers or other people. If a teacher has a problem, the child needs to know how to handle this situation without causing repercussions for themselves or the teacher.

The skill of assertiveness is very important to help children know the difference between being aggressive and assertive. Children will only get into trouble if they are overly aggressive without knowing when it is time to stop. They need to understand that aggression can take many forms, and you may have hurt someone's feelings by being aggressive towards them.

A child needs to know how to be assertive towards others so they don't hurt anyone else's feelings by not expressing what they want or need from others. This skill can also prevent a child from being cheated, taken advantage of, or bullied because they will be able to stand up for themselves when this happens.

A child needs to know how to accept responsibility for their mistakes, so they can learn from them and not repeat the same thing. This is an important skill because it helps children live up to their standards, feel valuable and needed in the world around them, have a sense of pride, and accomplish all the goals they set out for themselves. This will also help a child feel good about himself so that he will have a good sense of self-esteem and feel confident in all his decisions.

Children need to know how to listen to others, respect their opinions, and express their opinion in a way that will not hurt anyone else's feelings. These are the skills that children need to develop at a young age to get along with other people. This is especially important for parents because this will help them make the right decisions for their children.

This skill is important in life because it teaches children how to negotiate their own needs and goals with others. This skill can prevent a child from being taken advantage of by others because they will be able to stand up for themselves against bullying and exploitation at home and in school. If a child doesn't have this skill, they will always let people take advantage of them and not be able to stand up on their behalf.

This skill is important so that children can be assertive when they need to be and not have to worry about hurting others' feelings. This skill gives children the ability to take things by themselves without being aggressive and without having a fear of being punished for how they act.

This skill is very important in life because it teaches children how to listen to their own needs, wants, and goals in life so they can feel overall confident about themselves. They will know when it is time for them to do things for themselves so that they don't have problems with others or other people cheating them. This will also help them feel good about themselves and accomplish all the goals they set out for themselves in life.

Children need to know how to monitor their behavior and be able to control it. If a child does not have this skill, they may inadvertently end up hurting others' feelings by being overly aggressive or in other ways. They will also be unable to hold onto their self-esteem because they will always feel like they let people down because they cheated or acted without thinking first.

This skill is very important because it will help children feel good about themselves and accomplish all the goals they set out for themselves in life. Children need to know that if they make mistakes, then everyone makes mistakes, and no one is perfect, so they don't have to worry about this happening.

Children need to know how to let go of their fears, avoid making mistakes and learn from them. If they do not know this skill, they will waste a lot of time in their lives attempting to achieve things they don't want if they are afraid of failing. They won't be able to learn a lesson from their mistakes and will always feel like a failure.

Interpersonal effectiveness is important to children because it teaches them how to get along with others, stand up for themselves and care for their own needs. This helps build confidence in children and helps build a sense of self-esteem within them.

This is important in life because it teaches people how to make decisions based on how others feel about the situation. If someone feels very strongly about something, then the person making the decision needs to consider how this person feels about their own decision. This skill will help people understand how others feel about a situation and help them decide what is best for everyone involved.

This is an important skill to have in life because it teaches children how to feel good about themselves and accomplish all their goals in life. This will help them have a better sense of their self-esteem and feel confident in the decisions they make for themselves.

This skill is important for children because it teaches them strong decision-making skills based on what other people think about the situation. If someone feels very strongly about something, then this person needs to consider how this person feels about their decision before making any final decisions. This will help people understand how others feel about a situation and help them decide what is best for everyone involved in a difficult situation.

1.   8.Distress Tolerance Skills

Distress tolerance skills are ways to cope with distressing thoughts and feelings. They are skills that may be helpful to decrease the intensity of distress and associated physical symptoms or to change perspective on an event so that it is no longer as distressing.

Distress tolerance skills are a way for children to manage their emotions and react to situations in a healthy, positive manner. These skills can help children cope with stress, disappointment, and other challenging events. Tears are common reactions when children face challenges or difficult feelings. But, children need to learn healthy ways to cope with upsetting situations.

Here are some examples of distress tolerance skills:

1. Cognitive Restructuring

Cognitive restructuring is a distress tolerance skill that helps children change how they think about a situation. For example, a child who feels scared because he isn't as good as his friends at some sport might be encouraged to think about how much he practices and how hard he tries. He could then recognize that trying his best is important and can help him improve at sports. Encouraging the child to recognize something positive might help decrease his feelings of disappointment or sadness.

2. Distraction Skills

Distraction skills are ways to help children redirect their attention when they are upset. Children can often feel better if they can have a break from the situation. For example, a child crying because his friend was unkind might be encouraged to take on another activity, like getting a snack, reading a book, or playing outside. A distraction might help him feel better because it will distract him from the upsetting event or thought. Distraction skills are a way for children to change their focus and take action when they need to.

3. Predictability

Children often feel anxiety, sadness, or other negative emotions when uncertain about what will happen next. Children can reduce their negative emotions by practicing strategies to predict how events will unfold. For example, a child worried about going to school in the morning might be encouraged to get ready for bed the night before. This way, he knows that he has already done part of his routine and will have a better idea of how much time he has left.

4. Acceptance

Behavioral techniques (e.g., relaxation and deep breathing) are an excellent way to manage strong emotions and disturbing thoughts. Once the child learns new skills or develops greater emotional awareness, they will be better able to do things differently. Acceptance might help a child handle difficult emotions, especially when the child realizes that these emotions are natural and not a sign of something wrong.

5. Reappraisal

Reappraisal is a distress tolerance skill that helps children recognize how they think or feel. It can help them change how they see themselves or their situations. For example, a sad child might be encouraged to notice that he has lots of friends and gets upset because it's difficult to let them all down. Using the reappraisal skill, children will learn to develop more realistic expectations and avoid getting upset just because they don't always get what they want.

6. Decision-making Skills

Decision-making skills are techniques that help a child recognize how they think and act in situations. For example, if a child is frustrated with a friend who doesn't return messages, she might be encouraged to take some time alone and think about what she would want the friend to do next. She can then practice asking questions and looking for signs that the friend is trying to call her back.

7. Active Coping Strategies

Active coping strategies are methods used to manage stressful emotions and distressing thoughts so that they don't escalate into more intense emotions or disturbing thoughts. In these ways, active coping can help children find ways to continue being useful and useful to others. For example, a child who is frustrated about not being able to finish a paper might be encouraged to do some other task and think later about how to revise the paper. It might become more intense if she were told to take care of her disappointment immediately.

8. Positive Communication

Children often feel out of control, helpless, or frightened when they don't have the skills to express their feelings and ideas. By using positive communication skills, children can decrease their negative emotions and gain more control over how they think and act. Here are some examples of positive communication:

a) Valued Conversations

Valued conversations are ways that children can learn to recognize what they need and develop skills that will help them to manage difficult feelings (e.g., anger) in productive ways. This involves identifying supportive people (e.g., parents, teachers) and learning how to express their thoughts about difficult events or situations healthily.

b) Positive Reinforcement

Positive reinforcement is an effective way for children to change their behaviors. Positive reinforcement is a type of behavior that has a pleasant result and encourages the child to keep performing this behavior. For example, positive reinforcement might be giving a child stickers or an extra treat after he completes his homework. This will encourage the child to practice being responsible and make good choices regarding school work.

c) Mutual Help

Mutual help is another way that children can develop skills that will help them handle feelings of anxiety or distress healthily. By learning ways to talk about feelings and sharing difficult feelings with others, children can feel supported, cared for, and better able to cope with stress in productive ways.

d) Empathy Development

Empathy is taking someone else's perspective and putting themselves in their shoes. Empathy can help children develop skills that will allow them to cope with anxiety in productive ways. For example, a child who feels sad when his friend moves away might be encouraged to think about how his friend might feel or ask someone else if they can give him some information about how the friend feels on moving day. By developing empathy, children will become more likely to handle emotional suffering in healthy ways and be more aware of other people's feelings.

e) Persuasion Skills

Persuasion skills are techniques that help children ask for what they need. These techniques allow a child to learn how to give others an idea of what they need without becoming frustrated or too distressed. For example, a child might be encouraged to think about someone with similar feelings and how she healthily managed her feelings. She might then be encouraged to look for methods to help her deal with the situation.

9. Prosocial Skills

Prosocial skills are learned behaviors related to being helpful to other people. Prosocial skills are important for children because they can help them form attachments and shape their relationships with others. These skills can help many children have secure relationships with others, especially their parents or caregivers. The following are some examples of prosocial (i.e., helpful) behaviors:

a) Attachment-based Coping Skills

Attachment-based coping skills are ways that a child can develop new ways of thinking about emotional difficulties and experiences that will help them meet the needs of others. For example, a child with difficulty with schoolwork might be encouraged to find out where she is weak and how she can work on it. This will help her gain more confidence and knowledge about her strengths and weaknesses in school.

b) Self-management Skills

Self-management skills are ways that a child can learn to develop control over their own emotions, thoughts, and behaviors. Children can feel less anxiety or distress by learning how to think about difficult situations in productive ways. For example, if a child is angry and feels like shouting, he might be encouraged to take some deep breaths instead. This will allow him to think about what he needs to do next and let his frustration decrease on its own.

10. Breathing/relaxation

Breathing and relaxation are simple techniques for helping children to cope with situations that cause them stress. For example, if your child is feeling nervous about a test, they might imagine him or herself taking deep breaths to calm down and focus on the exam. In addition, you could ask them to tell you everything they need to do to concentrate on the exam while focusing on their breathing.

11. Identifying repetitive thoughts

Reinforcing kids to ask themselves if they are impatient or anxious can help them recognize their overreactions to situations. For example, when a child feels stressed, they might think they will fail the test. They might feel even more stressed because they thought they would fail the test. This frustrates them and makes them worry even more about failing the test. If your child notices that they are starting to worry about something (e.g., they're starting to feel frustrated, angry, nervous) and can identify that he's feeling these emotions, they might be better able to control them.

12. The calm down corner

A calm down corner is an area in the home where your child can go when they are feeling stressed to do some calming activities to relax their body and mind. Some ideas for the calm down corner might include: putting on soft music, writing about their feelings and thoughts in a journal, playing with a stress ball, reading a book, taking deep breaths (possibly with a partner), looking at calming pictures/posters/paintings on the wall (e.g., beach scenes), etc.

13. Developing a schedule and routine

Having a schedule and routine can help children to know what to expect in the day. They can also become more consistent with their thinking and feeling. If your child has developed routines (e.g., going to bed, waking up on time), they might be less likely to feel nervous or worried about things (e.g., he's going to be late if he doesn't wake up on time). In addition, it might reduce stress when they do not have control over what happens (i.e., stress about getting ready for school).

Children must learn how to deal with emotions to develop emotional intelligence. Children can help themselves by identifying their own emotions and learning how to cope with them. Although children may not be able to avoid stress, they can learn skills that allow them to tolerate it.

Developing emotional intelligence is an important part of becoming a resilient adult. Emotional intelligence can help children decide whether certain situations are stressful for them and teach them how to cope with such situations as well as others (e.g., being in a new school). Emotional intelligence can also help children figure out others' feelings, behaviors, and thinking styles, which can help them know what others need from them. Emotional intelligence can also help children be aware of their feelings, behaviors, and thinking styles, which can help them use that information to make decisions. Parents can develop emotional intelligence through a variety of activities with their children.

Awareness of one's feelings is the first step towards developing emotional intelligence. Parents should ask children questions that allow them to express different feelings. This will show children how they are feeling and allow them to figure out what they are feeling. For example, asking your child questions such as "How do you feel when you lose your toy?" may give them a better understanding of their emotions.

Children need to observe others and their situations to develop emotional intelligence. For example, you can ask your child to tell you how people are feeling in a picture or show them videos of others' behavior and what they are thinking. This will help your child to understand that others can feel different ways, just like they do.

Children also need an opportunity to practice skills that may help them cope with difficult situations. For example, when children lose their toy, they may become frustrated by this action (e.g., they yell at the other child who took it). This situation might give them a better understanding of how they feel when something bad happens.

Distress tolerance skills are essential to developing to cope with anxiety effectively. These skills are important because they allow children to learn how to handle distress, pain, and strong emotions using self-help techniques. Children who can tolerate distress might be better able to handle anxiety and distress. These skills also help children find support from others without becoming dependent on them. This can allow children to know how to get help for themselves when they need it. By learning distress tolerance skills, children are better able to develop self-care activities and coping skills. These coping skills will help children become healthier, happier, and more productive.

How to support your child

Children under five cannot verbally communicate their feelings or experiences. You might wonder how you can understand your child's emotions if they do not know how to express them verbally. Learning to understand your child's emotions is a way for you, as a parent or caregiver, to provide support for them effectively. Understanding your child's emotions means that you can help your child cope with strong feelings in healthy ways (e.g., crying when upset instead of being aggressive). You can learn to attend to your child's emotions in many ways.

Here are some examples of how you can learn about your child's emotions:

1. Counting and labeling feelings

One way that parents can learn to be aware of their children's feelings is by asking them questions or counting and labeling feelings with the help of their children. This can help your child learn to label and talk about their feelings. For example, you might ask your child to tell you how they feel by saying, "I'm happy" or "I'm mad." It is important to remember that children may not always be able to give you a clear answer. If your child feels scared, they might say he's a little scared instead of telling you what makes him feel scared. Asking questions about feelings is a way for parents and children to work together so that the child learns about their emotions and communicates them effectively.

2. Share experiences

Another way to understand your child's emotions is to share their experiences. Listening to your child's stories or thoughts can help you better understand their feelings about their own experiences. In addition, you might tell your child stories about how you felt when similar things happened to you. This lets him feel connected because he can understand how someone else has felt and experience something similar to him.

3. Be aware of your own emotions

Awareness of your own emotions is also important for parents to learn more about their children's emotions and provide effective support. Some signs that you might be having strong emotions include talking very quietly, feeling like crying, feeling sick to your stomach, sweating, and shaking. Becoming aware of your own emotions can help you identify what is going on for you so that you can provide support for your child. Being aware of your own emotions will also help increase the quality of your relationship with other people and give you a new perspective on stressful situations.

4. Be empathetic

Empathy is a way to understand how someone else feels (e.g., how someone's feelings make them feel) and guesses how they are feeling based on the context of their situation (e.g., reading cues such as facial expressions). Being empathetic is an important way to support your child. For example, if you empathize with your child by asking him why he feels sad, you might be able to understand how he feels and show him that you are there to help.

5. Encourage new coping skills

Encouraging your child's development of new coping skills is a way to help them learn skills they can use in the future (e.g., ways to handle sadness). When children do not have effective ways of dealing with their emotions, they can become upset in more brutal ways (e.g., becoming angry or anxious). Asking your child to draw or write about their feelings is a way to help develop creative ways of expressing feelings. This will help your child learn how to manage their emotions. It can also be helpful because it might show them how to express difficult situations productively.

Supporting your child's emotional development and coping skills is one of the best things you can do for them to become resilient. Asking your child questions to express their emotions will allow them to feel connected with you and others and improve their overall mood.

Distress tolerance skills are ideal for children with an oversensitivity to distress and difficulty staying emotionally regulated. Distress tolerance skills can help a child to manage intense feelings and stop him from engaging in behaviors that are not ideal for his development or emotional problems. To manage their emotions, children often need skills that help them to recognize feelings and thoughts for what they are. For example, children need to recognize that they are feeling nervous, frustrated, or sad to take the appropriate action. In addition, children need the skills to identify what thoughts distract them from the situation. Once children learn to recognize and acknowledge their feelings and thoughts for what they are, they can learn to develop various strategies to best deal with them. Children need to learn how to regulate their emotions. Effective strategies such as breathing, relaxing their muscles, and focusing on their breathing can help a child to feel calmer and more focused in the situation.

1.   9.Emotional Regulation Skills

One of the main skills in dialectical behavioral therapy is emotional regulation. Emotional regulation is how a person manages emotions' intensity, duration, frequency, and complexity. When an individual's emotional regulation skills are on point, they can control their emotions in times of stress or high emotion, so they do not experience negative effects. These skills help kids understand and manage their emotions. The emotional regulation skills in dialectical behavioral therapy will help kids understand their emotions, how to name them, and how to respond to them.

The following are Emotional regulation skills for children:

1. Identifying the Emotion

To understand and manage their emotions, kids need to know what they are feeling. First, help the child recognize that they are feeling an emotion. For example, when a child is sad, ask them:

Explain that emotions can come and go. Emotions are like weather patterns. Sometimes you feel happy, and other times you feel sad or angry. It's important to remember it's okay for kids to have these feelings and for them to come and go. Next, ask the child to identify which emotion they are feeling. This might require trial and error as naming emotions is a new skill for them. But keep trying and use examples from their daily life. For example, you can use these questions as a starting point:

If the child has difficulty identifying their feelings, help them focus on their physical feelings. Ask them if their heart is racing or if they feel the tension in their stomach. Also, ask about what their body parts are doing and how big or small those body parts feel. Make sure to affirm any emotions that the child does identify. For example:

When naming emotions, kids need to understand that there is not always one emotion that explains how we feel. Sometimes we feel happy and sad at the same time, or angry and afraid at different moments during the day or even within the same situation. It's important to teach the child that our emotions aren't always clear-cut.

2. Naming the Emotion

When kids can identify their emotions, they will begin to understand them better, and they will also begin to learn how they respond to different emotions. Help the child recognize that naming their feelings is an important step in managing their emotions. Ask them what they feel whenever an emotion comes up, and have them name it. When this becomes a habit, it will help the child realize that their feelings are okay and teach them about their emotional responses. If your child is having a hard time identifying what they are feeling, you can ask questions like:

-What is this feeling like?

-What does it look, sound, and taste like?

-What are the feelings and physical sensations in my body like?

-How can I name this feeling?

Once kids learn to identify and name their emotions, help them understand that the next step is labeling them. The child uses the word "I" when describing their emotional responses. For example:

When kids learn to label their emotions and understand that their emotions aren't always clear-cut, they will begin to be able to tell you about all of their feelings as they occur.

3. Responding to Emotions

The third step of emotional regulation is to learn how to respond to their emotions. There are three main ways that kids learn how to respond:

A. By reacting: When kids notice that they have a certain emotion, they may begin to act in ways that cause the intensity of their feeling to increase even more. The way we have been trained since childhood, however, is for us to act in ways that make the intensity less intense and for us to avoid these situations altogether if we have the opportunity. Dialectical Behavioral Therapy (DBT) teaches children how this has led them down a destructive path regarding their relationships and life choices.

B. By avoiding: When kids react to their emotions in a less than productive way, they may resort to avoiding those situations that cause them to feel certain emotions. No doubt this has been the pattern for them up until this point. DBT teaches kids how to manage their emotions and respond in ways that help them improve relationships and make healthy choices about how they live their lives.

C. By accepting: When kids learn to accept their emotional responses, they can better manage those emotions. Acceptance will further decrease the intensity of their emotional responses. This is a skill that many adults struggle with, so it isn't a skill that children will pick up quickly or easily. DBT also teaches kids how to respond in ways that will help them build relationships, improve their quality of life, and create positive outlooks on the future.

4. Acting

The final step in emotional regulation is to learn to act in ways that are not only going to decrease the intensity of their feelings but also it's going to increase the way they feel about themselves. Many kids who have been taught that emotions are bad to have learned how to express those emotions negatively. Even kids taught to express their emotions appropriately tend not to do so successfully and still struggle with self-esteem issues.

The first step in communicating is for children to understand that they can use words when they are feeling angry. They have to learn that their words can be powerful tools.

A skill that will help kids learn how to communicate their needs and wants is learning the "I" message. The "I" message means that kids are using the word "I" when they are communicating with others instead of using the word "you." When kids use the "I" message, it also helps them take responsibility for their actions. This will make it easier for them to express what they need and blame others for their bad feelings (usually unproductive).

Another thing that kids need to learn how to do is to communicate their ideas and goals. When kids can communicate their ideas, they will begin to understand them better. I've seen over the years that when kids talk about what they want, it is often very different from what they mean. They don't realize it. Help them understand that they have to learn how to express what they mean instead of just talking about what they want. Having them practice saying what they mean will be a good and healthy way to begin managing their emotions.

A way to regulate emotions is to learn what causes the child to have certain moods and how they could change their mood if it makes them feel worse. For instance, some kids might be more likely to yell when they are hungry or frustrated, while others might yell after being praised or when they are feeling very excited by something. The important thing for your child to remember is that the more different emotions you name and the more times you can recognize them, the more skill you will have to regulate them. This will help them understand their feelings and how they can reduce their negative reactions when they feel certain emotions.

One of the ways to regulate your emotional state is to remember that adults see your feelings as well, but sometimes their actions do not make sense. A kid might think no one will see their feelings if they yell or cry. This is untrue, as adults sometimes notice a kid's feelings and react accordingly. If a child is being reprimanded for crying after spilling his milk, the child might think that crying is not a good idea. While this could be true at the moment, the child might not realize that it was frustration over spilling their milk that made them cry. In this case, the child can learn to regulate their emotions by thinking about how they would feel if they were upset at something and someone got mad at them for being upset and did nothing to help fix their problem. For example, the child might tell themselves that they would feel ashamed and angry at seeing someone get upset when they could do something to help fix the problem. The child might also find it useful to think about how a friend would respond when they cried because they felt embarrassed by something. This might help get them out of thinking that all crying is bad and wrong.

When you are angry, frustrated, or sad, it is important to try and find a way to express these negative emotions in some way other than yelling or crying. One better option for children with trouble regulating their emotions is writing about them. I recommend that children who struggle with emotions write about their feelings in a journal. It may also be helpful for you to write about what you are feeling and why you feel that way. Writing down your feelings can help you better understand them and find ways to control them. It is also important for kids to learn how to express themselves in other ways. Another way for kids to do this is by talking with a family member or friend about their feelings. This can be very helpful during times of stress and anger as well as sadness due to the death of a loved one, divorce, or other stressful situations that the child is facing at home or school.

Another important skill in emotional regulation is to be a good listener. If your child learns to listen, it will help them understand their feelings and those of others. This will allow them to have the ability to process what they are thinking and feeling from both their own and other people's perspectives. If your child can do this, it will also help them regulate their emotions better.

One way that kids try and control their emotions is by having someone read their stories on what they might be feeling. Reading them a story may help them realize that they are not the only person feeling this way and may also help them understand how to deal with those feelings. When a child feels that they are the only one who can't control their emotions, it can devastate their self-esteem. Showing your child how to regulate their emotions can make them feel better about themselves and better deal with any emotional distress they might feel.

Little children, who tend to have a harder time regulating their emotions, can be given a small toy car as a gift, allowing them to learn how to control it as they age. Younger children, who may not be able to control their emotions to the extent that older kids and adults can,

can be given a piece of paper with future pictures. This paper is a picture of the child when they are older and has improved at controlling their emotions. Pictures of them achieving goals will help them feel more confident about themselves as they grow up.

Another way for a child to learn how to manage their emotions is to draw a picture of what they are feeling and then write the emotion in some way on the picture. This will help them understand their emotions and allow them to cope with those emotions. It can also be helpful for them to have someone explain to them how they feel so that they can understand themselves better.

If your child is having problems regulating their emotions at home, school, or with other kids, there are some things you can do at home. The first thing to do is find out what drives your child's negative feelings. If your child is having difficulty at school, try to figure out why. If it is because of bullying by other kids, find out if there is something the teacher can do to stop it. It may also help your child find someone they can talk with about their feelings. This way, they can get their feelings and emotions out in the open and not keep them bottled up inside, where they will cause problems later on. Another good thing you can do at home is to engage in activities that force your child into experiencing positive emotions. This way, when your child has a negative emotion, they will be able to compare it to these positive emotions and realize that negative emotions aren't so bad.

1.   10.Cognitive Skills

Cognitive skills are the ability to think and problem-solve. They are the skills we use daily to make decisions and understand our experiences. Cognitive skills can also include understanding cause and effect to recognize a behavior's trigger or consequence. For example, the person might yell and hit if a scary or upsetting situation. It is difficult for a child to identify what happened and how to handle the situation without the ability to verbalize their feelings. They also use cognitive skills to understand cause and effect; if they are scared or upset, they do/say things that will upset/upset someone else. When children have difficulty with cognitive skills, it often affects their relationships with others. The following are examples of cognitive skills that a child can learn in DBT:

1. Anticipation and planning - Looking ahead and planning for what will happen next enable a person to be more successful. With this skill, a person can control impulsive behavior, minimize stress, and prioritize what needs to be done better. A child with poor cognitive skills might not think about how their actions or words will affect others or themselves. They might also have difficulty making decisions which can lead to impulsive action.

2. Problem-solving - assessing, identifying, and solving problems provides a safe and effective means of self-regulation. The child can use cognitive skills to change a problematic behavior or negative thought pattern. For example, if the child is feeling angry, they would identify it as a problem that they want to address. This skill also helps

children with depression recognize that they have a thought (to change the thought).

3. Organization - Being able to organize their thoughts and feelings and respond effectively is crucial, especially in the classroom. When a child has poor cognitive skills, it can be difficult to process information before responding, which usually results in impulsive behavior or failure at school.

4. Critical thinking - Thinking critically can help a person assess and evaluate their thoughts, emotions, behavior, and circumstances. It also empowers a person to decide how to handle certain circumstances or situations. This skill helps the child make good choices and take healthy risks.

5. Self-awareness - A good look in the mirror allows people to become more in tune with their thoughts, feelings, and behaviors. This can help them recognize what they need to improve and what they do well. It helps them become more self-aware, which is the first step to addressing unhealthy behavior patterns.

Cognitive skills can be improved with DBT skills practice for a person to make more positive choices. Several techniques used through DBT help people develop these skills by learning new ways of thinking about the world. Skills training is an area of intensive therapy that helps improve cognitive skills. These skills are taught in a structured way for the participant to learn and practice using skills.

DBT skills can include learning new ways of thinking about situations and problems, problem-solving, making decisions, increasing positive behaviors, and balancing emotions. Some skills are about being able to talk about one's feelings in a new way. Some cognitive skill-building ideas can include: how to solve problems without fighting, how to make decisions that feel good rather than ones that will cause conflict, how to talk with people so they will listen and understand what you are saying or how to figure out if someone is right or wrong.

Several different exercises can be used for cognitive skill training. The emphasis is on figuring things out, how to solve problems peacefully and how to talk with people to foster understanding and cooperation. For example, the person might talk about a time when they felt angry and then try to think of ways to solve the problem, so it doesn't get out of hand. They may then discuss how they were successful in solving problems by preventing a fight or how they were not successful.

Developing Cognitive Skills in Kids:

There are several ways in which a parent can help their child develop cognitive skills:

1. Talking and reading to the child regularly, as early as possible, will help develop language and interest in books. This will assist in developing vocabulary and communication skills and the emotional bonds formed while reading together.

2. Help the child to understand their emotions and how to express them appropriately. This will help develop several aspects of social

interaction, such as empathy and perspective-taking, which are essential for good mental health.

3. Encourage creative play in free-choice activities such as art, music, dance, story-telling, or writing. These activities will help the child engage the imagination and develop cognitive skills that may not be addressed in school but can still be helpful for success in school and life.

4. Help children to cope with stress by encouraging them to use cognitive skills such as planning or problem-solving when faced with situations that may cause stress.

5. Encourage the child to practice cognitive skills in school. This could include reading aloud, sharing work with classmates, and practicing math skills such as number changes, addition, and subtraction.

6. Help the child develop the social skills to interact with others in a non-abusive way. These may include assertiveness, self-control, emotional management, or empathy. Recognizing their feelings and staying focused on tasks is essential for success at school or in life.

7. Encourage the child to develop a daily routine or schedule to help with self-regulation.

8. Encourage the child to set goals for themselves, such as academic goals, healthy behaviors (exercise/eating a balanced diet/sleeping well), or career goals (to become recognized in their field).

9. Help the child understand their strengths and weaknesses and how they can work on the weakest areas to improve their performance in school and life.

10. Have patience! Just because you have struggled with these skills in the past doesn't mean your children need to struggle; some people learn differently than others.

Cognitive skills are essential for developing positive relationships. Researchers have found that self-efficacy was most strongly related to children's emotional and behavioral adjustment and academic achievement. According to this research, children who have good cognitive skills are more likely to have good relationships with their parents and teachers, which will enhance their learning experience

Children with cognitive difficulties often struggle socially. The impact on peer relationships can be considerable. Poor social skills may cause the child to receive less socially acceptable treatment from peers than children without these problems. Additionally, they may be unable to plan because they cannot accurately read others' intentions or feelings. This can lead to poor choices, which then may escalate and intensify. These difficulties can lead to emotional and behavioral problems such as aggression, bullying, and withdrawal. These examples highlight the importance of working on children's cognitive skills.

The long-term effects of poor cognitive skills can be devastating. The child is often unable to learn effectively and cannot manage their emotions well. This can lead to lifelong struggles with peer relationships, academic success, employment, promotion, and social interaction, which are important for a healthy life.

Children's cognitive skills seem to be linked with the ability to self-regulate negative emotions. Children with poor self-regulation were more likely to have problems adjusting in school, either academically or behaviorally. Self-regulation is associated with better reading ability in adolescents and increased social competence and empathy. Those with the greater cognitive ability also have better self-control and can control impulses more effectively. There is evidence that this relationship is mediated by the parietal lobe, which controls the ability to keep track of time and plan in advance. The relationship between the parietal lobe and self-regulation has been directly demonstrated in children and adults.

Those with low cognitive skills are less likely to develop and maintain healthy social relationships, which can be essential to mental health. It has been shown that those with poor cognitive skills have difficulty achieving good relationships with their friends, a factor that is strongly linked to mental health.

Research indicates that children who can regulate their emotions effectively can more easily put cognitive functioning into action through emotional intelligence techniques. This means that children who can better regulate their emotions tend to have more developed cognitive skills, such as analysis, planning, and decision-making.

Those with low cognitive skills often struggle in school, particularly in areas where they must apply higher-order thinking skills.

Benefits of Cognitive skills for Kids:

Cognitive skills have several benefits. The following are some of the most important ones:

1. Better academic performance:

Studies have found that children who can think more analytically and with greater creativity in math and writing tend to perform better academically. The ability to organize and analyze problems is also associated with improvements in reading, especially for those struggling with reading difficulties.

2. Increased self-esteem:

Those with better cognitive skills tend to feel more confident about their performance at school or home. They also tend to be more aware of their capabilities, emotions, and behaviors.

3. Higher self-control:

Good cognitive skills lead to greater self-control, better social competence, and fewer behavioral problems. Children who are better at controlling their impulses tend to have fewer conduct problems and are better able to handle stressful situations. Those who can control their emotions tend to be more popular and do better socially than those who do not have these skills.

4. Better social skills:

Children with poor cognitive skills often struggle socially. Those who can regulate their emotions in ways others find acceptable will have an easier time making friends and interacting well with others.

5. Improved sleep patterns:

Parents have reported that children with good cognitive skills tend to have better sleep patterns, including falling asleep more easily and remaining asleep longer. These children also have fewer nightmares than those with lower cognitive abilities.

6. Self-awareness:

The ability to think about one's thinking is associated with increased self-awareness, leading to better problem-solving and more insight into one's emotions and motivations. Those who can accurately reflect on themselves tend to be more empathetic toward others and make decisions that are in their best interests. They also feel greater control over their lives and how they operate in the world.

7. Better mental health:

Those with good cognitive skills are more likely to be able to regulate their emotions in ways that others will find acceptable. This is associated with higher self-esteem and better social relationships, which are important for good mental health.

8. Greater creativity:

Creativity is an essential part of the thinking process, and all children need time away from immediate demands to develop their unique thoughts and ideas. Cognitive aides such as thinking and imagination can be helpful when working on projects or solving problems. Still, they impede success when the situation requires immediate action or reaction.

Cognitive Skills are very much useful to a child's development. This is because they can think logically and critically, which helps them solve problems and deal with social pressure constructively. These skills also enhance a child's well-being by helping them regulate their emotions and thoughts.

Cognitive skills are developed by reading, writing, puzzles, and critical thinking. These skills can be applied to schoolwork, including math, science, and language arts. Kids who process information analytically will often have the highest cognitive scores. This can greatly improve the child's academic performance in school, resulting in higher self-esteem and better social relationships with peers. Children who have been properly taught cognitive skills in the early years of their lives will most likely develop these skills. This can be accomplished by parents and caregivers teaching the child how to learn and use their environment, including their senses, to improve their cognitive development. Cognitive skills are important to early childhood development because they affect the child's development in both academic and social areas. By developing cognitive skills in a child, parents can help them deal with their problems maturely and think of new ways to solve or understand a problem.

Children with good cognitive skills may face difficulties later in life in school or social situations. But by using emotional intelligence techniques to regulate these emotions, children can better control themselves and cope with stressful situations later in life. As a result, the child will grow up strong and feel confident about their abilities.

1.   11.Living Skills

Living skills are self-administered skills that help children with their daily life. These skills allow your child to know what they are doing and how they feel. They also provide opportunities for your child to think about the world around them and to use their imagination, which is an important part of learning new things. This is an individualized skill that can be taught and practiced regularly. These skills are:

Listening, understanding, and responding to others' needs. This includes taking someone's turn and listening when someone is talking to them. Children with autism can struggle with this, as they may not respond appropriately when children or adults are asking for their turn or just not paying attention at all. There are many ways your child can be taught to listen appropriately, including listening with the eyes and hands and singing songs to encourage kids to listen attentively. Some children will not be able to pay attention while on the activities board, so it is a good idea to incorporate other ways children can learn how to listen by themselves.

Problem-solving: This includes teaching your child how to plan and make decisions. Many kids with autism have difficulty planning and making decisions. They may not know how to start or finish a project or need help problem-solving simple daily tasks. The problem-solving process is important because it helps children learn how to break problems down into smaller parts that are easier to solve. Children will learn how to handle difficult situations, such as when they don't know what to say or do in a particular situation. They can also use problem-solving when they have trouble doing something they want (but cannot complete).

Interacting with others: This skill involves social skills and is invaluable for children with autism. Interacting positively will help your child be more comfortable in social situations. It is important that your child understand non-verbal communication and how to use these skills appropriately to communicate effectively. This can be done by modeling appropriate behavior, watching other children interact while role-playing, or working on conversations with a speech therapist or coach. Interacting skillfully can help make a big difference in how your child feels during social interactions (e.g., play dates).

Coordination of body movements: Coordination involves fine motor skills, eye contact, and the ability to follow directions on paper or through the computer application program. Your child will learn how to groom, dress, and bathe by themselves. They may not be able to put on a shirt or tie their shoes all by themselves, but your child can still learn how to do these things. Coordination of body movements also requires children to know what body parts go where and when. This can help children communicate with others through eye contact or gestures. You can teach your child ways to interact with family members or toys by slowly moving different parts of their bodies that they may not be able to express when they are alone (e.g., using facial expressions like nodding or shaking).

Negotiation: Negotiation involves recognizing other people's feelings and needs through actions, words, and facial expressions. When your child learns to negotiate, they will learn more about how other children feel about their actions. They also need to learn how to express their feelings, needs, and wants. Kids with autism often have trouble expressing their feelings about things happening around them or to them. When a reward system is in place (e.g., sticker charts), children can learn how to use negotiation skills to ask for things they want and help friends when problems arise. Negotiation can be difficult at first, but as your child ages, they will learn more about how to use this skill and become more proficient.

Interpreting non-verbal communication (body language): This is important to help children understand what other people think or feel by reading facial expressions and body language. Before teaching this skill, children must first be taught how to read someone's face. Children can learn how to read faces by looking at photographs of different facial expressions and writing what the person might be feeling in a journal. They can also practice making the different facial expressions and identify them with the pictures from their journal. As they learn to read faces, they will be able to recognize the different expressions.

When children learn to interpret non-verbal communication, they need to use their brains differently. They must learn to focus on the person rather than just the face. When people are talking, they might not be able to make out what is being said, and study strategies can be used to help children understand what people are saying. For example, you can have your child repeat back words or phrases you have said in your own words. If your child does not know what certain things mean, they should listen and not ask questions, so they will have time to read the expression on other people's faces and figure out what they mean before asking questions. Listening to non-verbal communication is important for all children to learn, so you will want to work on this skill as often as possible with your child.

Journals, social stories, and visual schedules are great ways to help your child build their listening and problem-solving skills. You can write in the journal what your child likes and dislikes and how they wish people would react when they do things that are not socially acceptable. These journals should be read out loud every night while you bathe your child or before falling asleep at night. You can put pictures of things they like and stickers on the things they want. You can also create a daily schedule at bedtime and ask your child if they need to be woken up or if they need to use the bathroom, etc. These techniques will help foster young children's listening, problem-solving and social skills.

Another great way to help your child learn how to solve problems is through a puppet. You can use a puppet to model interactive play and help your child learn how to communicate better with others. The puppet can help your child interpret people's body language and facial expressions so they can learn about how other people feel and think about things happening around them. Puppets are also an effective way for children to practice their social skills. If your child is having trouble understanding what others mean when they talk or want something, you can have the puppet ask the person what they want or are feeling. That way, the person understands loud and clear.

Even though learning how to talk and have conversations is significant for your child when they are old enough, children should build their language skills early in life. Research has shown that children who speak at a very early age can often develop strong social skills or those who do not speak well are more likely to have lower levels of empathy. Young children learn language by listening to their parents' words, reading books, watching television, listening to music, and playing with other kids. They should be able to watch movies with subtitles that teach language and literacy while teaching social skills.

Laughter, music, and other sounds should help teach your child different words and phrases. When you hear something interesting to you, you will want to talk about it. You can use sounds such as animals or bird noises; they rarely come up in conversation with others and are a great way to help your child learn new words. If you hear a sound that your child does not recognize, explain it to them so they can have the opportunity to learn more about their surroundings. Activity schedules are another great tool because they provide a visual schedule that children can follow while learning new skills.

It is important for parents to spend time with their children, play games with them, and read to them. The more practice your child has with these skills, the better they will be able to concentrate and manage their feelings. In addition, be sure to provide a quiet space for your child when angry or upset so they can calm themselves down. If possible, make a safe space for them to go when they feel frustrated. Sometimes children need their own private space to calm down and get used to new things happening around them.

1.   12.Family Support

Family support is a key factor in Dialectical Behavioral Therapy (DBT). Kids thrive when a support system is around them, and DBT can help build that. It's not about providing 'patience' but being with your child for whatever life throws your way. As children grow up and need more independence, this usually means moving away from the family support structure of DBT and into the world. However, these skills learned from DBT can help your child in any social environment they find themselves in later in life. Skills taught in DBT are meant to help your child cope with life, no matter where they are or who they are with. The most important thing is to be there for them and guide them through the use of these skills.

Family support is key to a child's recovery from DBT. Even if the parents don't fully understand, they should be supportive and loving when their child learns and tries new skills, even if they don't work. Teaching DBT to a child when you don't understand it yourself is hard but not impossible. The most important thing is providing unconditional love for your child and for them to know that you will always be there no matter what.

As children grow and start to develop their own identities, it is important to help them understand who they are and give them the tools to help their personalities. This doesn't mean you can't express your own opinions, though. It's all about defining who you are and helping your child build a solid foundation upon which they can base the rest of their personality.

Ways through which family can support children in Dialectical Behavioral Therapy:

1. Be an advocate for your child.

Listen to your child, don't judge them, and provide unconditional love. Show them that you are there for them when they need you the most and that they can trust you with anything they have to say. This will keep them from bottling things up, a common characteristic among many children with anger problems. When they feel like they can't talk to you, they might be more likely to turn to things like drugs or alcohol as a way of dealing with their feelings.

2. Model the behaviors and skills taught in Dialectical Behavioral Therapy.

If your child is learning new skills, they need to be able to see you using them as well. This will help them better understand how these skills work and show them that they are effective and possible to use in real-life situations.

3. Give your child the tools to solve problems.

Instead of judging your child for their actions, help them understand that they have choices to make. This will help them build a stronger sense of self and give them something to work with when they aren't feeling themselves. When they overcome challenges, they can feel more confident and deal with life more effectively.

4. Don't forget to let your child be a kid.

While DBT is meant to help your child learn better ways to deal with life, it doesn't mean you can't still let them do things that will help them feel more like kids. If they want to play video games and watch cartoons, allow them. This allows you to spend time alone with them and keeps them from thinking about the things going on in their life. This is important, especially when they come home from school and feel like they have no escape from the difficulties they face in day-to-day life.

5. Keep communication open.

The parent needs to know how their child feels and what's going on in their life. This might be a good time to discuss what they are learning in DBT so they can have some support when needed. Even if they don't agree with your child's actions, it is important to have an open and honest understanding. By doing this, you will gain an ally against them instead of helping them become disconnected from what is happening in their life.

6. Allow your child a chance to express themselves.

As kids get older and start to learn how to express themselves, they need to be able to do so without the fear of judgment. They must realize that no one will judge them and that everything will be alright, even if their actions aren't exactly 'normal.' They also need to realize that communication is important and try as hard as possible to make things work for everyone. In this case, it is good for them and you as well.

7. Be open-minded.

When your child is making mistakes, listening to them and understanding where they are coming from can be hard. It may make things easier for you if you try to think of another perspective and see situations from their point of view. This will allow you to understand the struggles they have in their life and will hopefully help you support them more effectively when it's necessary. The main thing is that you do what needs to be done for your child, not what makes the most sense. It is always important that children feel comfortable with their parents no matter what, and it's all about giving them enough support without micromanaging them.

8. Encourage self-examination.

Please encourage your child to examine themselves and their struggles regularly. This is important during any therapy, but especially during DBT. The skills taught in DBT must be used daily to be effective. Additionally, they must be used when required.

9. Remember that kids will always make mistakes and mess up at some point.

When we talk about 'tough love, we aren't talking about being harsh or cruel; rather, it's about giving your child what they need and not necessarily what you think they should have right now. If you have already made your child aware of the consequences of doing this, then it is up to them to decide if they would rather follow through or deal with the consequences. The important thing is that they are allowed to make a choice and that you are there for them no matter which decision they make.

Family support is essential for children facing any challenge, including anger issues. This is especially true for DBT, and everyone in the family must understand what is happening. The more you can understand your child's behaviors, the better equipped you will be to help them overcome their problems. When things cannot be worked out in therapy, it will fall on you to provide support until such a resolution can be found.

Doing this might seem difficult initially, but with a little practice and patience, it becomes second nature over time. It's very important to remember that no one person can provide all of the support for your child, though you can always play a crucial role in helping them overcome life's challenges.

It's very tough to see your child go through these struggles but make it a point to continue providing support. When you do this, you will be able to help them overcome their problems and feel less alone, both of which are important for a child's development.

1. 13.The Group Is a Vehicle To Change

Group therapy can effectively change your behavior because it provides many opportunities to learn different ways of solving problems and handling difficult situations. A group allows children to practice new behaviors with people they trust who understand what they have been through.

Working in groups also helps children feel less alone and more connected to others. In many ways, working in a group can be the same as working independently. In a highly structured setting such as a residential treatment program, a group may be the only place where behavior change is encouraged.

In any group therapy situation, a trained therapist works with the group members to help them learn how to use their strengths and deal with any personal issues they face. The therapist helps set ground rules for the group and ensures that every group member understands them. The therapist also tries to help group members learn how to resolve conflicts while allowing each person their point of view.

Children will be given many opportunities to practice new skills and behaviors in a group setting. Group members are often asked to take turns discussing their problems and working through them. Their group members will act as mirrors, reflecting your strengths and weaknesses. The therapist will often play the role of coach or observer, asking questions to keep the discussion focused on important issues. There will also be resources for listening and support when times are difficult for them.

Children benefit from group therapy because children have often not had the opportunity to interact with other children. Group therapy can help break down their isolation. It can also give them a better understanding of themselves, others, and the world around them.

Children who have experienced abuse or neglect may be extremely shy, mistrustful, or even hostile toward adults. Some may believe that adults are only interested in controlling or punishing them. Group therapy can help children overcome these feelings and develop a positive view of adults in their lives – parents and other teachers, counselors, therapists, and social service workers – as well as develop friendships with other group members.

A group offers a safe place for children to express themselves freely, allowing each child to be an equal member of the group. As children learn to trust others, they can begin to develop their solutions and solutions for problems in their individual lives.

Sometimes children who have been neglected or abused by a parent or other caregiver may feel that they cannot live up to the expectations of others. In group therapy, children can learn how to ask for what they want, show appreciation for others' help, and express feelings of sadness without fear of punishment. Children who can express themselves are more likely to grow into more self-confident adults who know how to deal with difficult life situations.

Often children who have been abused or neglected are afraid of becoming parents. Group therapy can help break down these feelings of shame and guilt. By helping the children feel confident about their parenting ability, group therapy allows them to learn how to be good parents even when they are not around their children.

Because many peer relationships are important for healthy development, group therapy often helps children make new friends who can help them deal with their feelings of loneliness and isolation. These new friendships often form the basis for a healthy support system that is available throughout life. Group therapy also allows these children to give and receive love without needing anyone's approval except themselves.

Because others have often punished children, group therapy offers them a safe place to express themselves and learn more effective ways of dealing with their emotions. Therapists often give children alternate forms of punishment, such as privileges, which they can earn when they meet certain goals or accomplish certain tasks.

Much research has shown that one of the most effective ways to treat children who have suffered from severe abuse and neglect is to support them in forming new friendships within a supportive community of other children who are also in recovery. Children feel better about themselves when they can be strong for others without being criticized or humiliated by an authority figure such as a parent. In group therapy, children gain experience helping and getting to know other children with similar problems. This gives them a sense of self-worth and leads to healthier adult relationships.

In group children can:

• Learn new ways of behaving in difficult situations when dealing with a problem.

• Talk about difficult subjects with other children who can relate to you.

• Feel less lonely and more connected to others through feeling more accepted by other children.

• Gain new friendships and learn how to develop relationships with adults.

• Express your feelings without fearing consequences from adults or peers in the group. This can help you feel happier and more confident about yourself.

• Learn how to interact with peers without frustration, anger, or anxiety. This can help you communicate better with your friends and family members as well as take on new challenges in your life outside the home, such as school, work, or college activities.

These groups provide safe opportunities to explore their feelings and values in an atmosphere where they feel accepted by the group members. Groups also provide a forum in which members can discuss their emotional reactions with one another. Group members are usually more thoughtful about what they say because they know it will impact others. They often come away from this experience with greater self-awareness and empathy for others' experiences.

For the children who attend these groups, this is the first time they have been held accountable for their actions in a supportive and empathetic environment. Frequently, parents are shocked at how much their children understand about themselves and others. As a result, many become more confident as they develop close friendships.

The positive effects of group therapy for children who have experienced abuse or neglect are often long-lasting. In a recent study, researchers found that child abuse survivors who had participated in groups in the past were more likely to make better decisions for their health and well-being than those who had not. When asked about the effects of groups, most participants reported that they felt calmer, more self-assured, and less self-critical than before. They also felt closer to their families and friends. For many, these new friendships served as valuable reminders that they were loved and did not need to fight with their parents any longer.

Group therapy helps children feel less alone and more connected to others, encouraging them to express their feelings more openly. When a child has been through hardship or abuse, it is important for them to feel accepted by others so that they will not feel as though they have to hide such things from others. The child feels like they belong and are a valuable group member. The child is also with other children who can relate to them and are going through similar life hardships.

Effective group therapy can also greatly impact a child's recovery. Since peer relationships are so important to psychological health, children who attend group therapy learn how to form healthy relationships with others. By helping the children learn how to relate with one another, they will be able to form healthy peer relationships and have better social skills as adults.

1.   14. Problem Solving Strategies

Problem-solving is a powerful way to understand and manage your emotions, thoughts, and behaviors. Problem-solving strategies can help your child solve problems when they feel stuck and frustrated.

Problem-solving is a skill that can benefit your child in future relationships and many daily situations.

Problem-solving is an important skill for children to learn and practice, so it's helpful to give your child many opportunities to practice it. You can help your child learn how to problem-solve in many ways. You can do some things yourself, while others you may want your child or other caregivers to do with them.

Your attitude drives the process, so ensure you are optimistic when sharing this information with others. You want the relationship between all parties involved in problem-solving (yourself, therapists, and counselors) to be positive and collaborative while maintaining a firm and authoritative stance.

Problem-solving begins with an issue. Your child may come to you with a problem, or you may offer to help them with their problem. Problem-solving is about finding solutions. Therefore, it's important to summarize the problem your child is experiencing. You should be asking, "What's wrong?" "What can we do?" "How would you like to solve this problem?"

It's important to devise a plan rather than just giving them advice. If you're only giving advice and not listening to their needs, you're probably not helping them solve the issue. Also, mental health professionals are trained in this behavior because it is how they can successfully help others.

It's also important not to give your child the answers or solutions. You must listen carefully to what they want and need. You can't truly understand their situation unless you listen carefully and allow them to speak openly about their thoughts and feelings. It would be best if you heard their words to be sure to use the right solution or answer.

You will want to find a way for your child to practice Problem-solving. They may need to practice their skills over and over before they get them right. There are also many times when children have trouble solving problems—they can't come up with good solutions, or they lose their temper, give up or resort to old behaviors that don't work. This is typical and very common.

The Problem-Solving Strategies below are a helpful guide in helping children learn how to solve problems themselves.

1. Identify the Problem

The first step in problem-solving is to identify the problem. Your child's feelings and thoughts and your observations of their behavior will help you identify the problem. You can also ask your child what they think the problem is. Make sure you summarize the problem as simply as possible and avoid jumping to conclusions about why your child is having a particular reaction.

Identifying problems is best where you won't be interrupted, such as in a quiet room or on an outing.

2. Brainstorm for Solutions

Once you have identified the problem, you can begin to brainstorm solutions. This is also a good time to ask your child what they think would be a good solution. Your child's solutions may differ from yours, so it's important to keep an open mind and respect their ideas. Also, be sure not to criticize or discourage their ideas. Think of all the possible solutions together, no matter how good or bad.

-Once you have brainstormed many possible solutions, you will begin to prioritize them and discuss which ones will work best.

-If you or your child gets stuck, try to think of how someone else might solve the problem.

-Keep in mind that some problems can't be solved, so there's nothing wrong with trying to live with it.

3. Take Action

Once you have considered all possible solutions, the next step is to take action and commit to doing something about the problem. You want your commitment to be as realistic as possible; don't make commitments that are too difficult or will take a long time to complete. When you take action, be sure it doesn't hurt others, and consider if others may get hurt due to taking action.

4. Evaluate Progress

As you go along, evaluate progress and ask your child what they think of the progress that has been made. This will allow them to share their feelings about the situation and help identify new problems. You'll also have a chance to adjust your plan based on information shared by your child.

5. Continue to Problem-Solve

This is the most important part of problem-solving because it will mean that you and your child can continue to solve problems together in the future. When you've finished problem-solving, ask your child how they would like to remember the experience. They may want to think about what went well or could be improved. If they have a final idea of something they'd like to improve, ensure you include them when it's time for action.

6. Ask for Help

If you find that your child needs help learning these strategies, make sure you ask for help from a professional who will be able to teach these skills to your child.

7. Review and Rehearse

You can review these strategies again at a later date. Think about which skills may need to be practiced more and plan to do that. You can also use role-playing or cartoon characters to help your child remember how to problem-solve.

Some children will feel a lot of anxiety about being able to problem solve on their own, so you must be there for them during this process until they are comfortable with these strategies.

Problem-solving is a useful skill that can be very useful in many situations. Your child must have an opportunity to practice problem-solving with you and other professionals that can help them. Learning how to problem solve with others will also help children learn how to solve their problems when others aren't around. It's important to help children learn how to problem solve and have an open mind that they may not be able to solve all problems.

Problem-solving is also a good tool for helping children develop self-esteem and confidence in their ability to deal with difficult situations. The more your child practices these skills, the more confident they will become and the better problem-solver they'll be.

Problem-solving is a life skill that is very important in helping children cope with stressful situations and emotions. If your child has trouble with problem-solving, try using the above strategies to help your child understand how to solve problems.

These problem-solving strategies are essential skills that are vital to develop and practice. They will help your child learn to solve problems independently and teach them to be more responsible, respectful, and caring of others. Problem-solving skills will help your child in many different ways throughout their life. By practicing these problem-solving skills, children will be able to take responsibility and learn how to solve problems when they occur later in life. It ultimately helps them become more independent and confident in the long term.

Conclusion

Dialectical Behavioral Therapy is useful for children and adolescents of all ages. It's used to help children and adolescents learn how to regulate their emotions and behaviors, develop relationships, and make positive choices in the face of adversity.

It's best suited for children with chronic problems with intense emotions, impulsive behaviors, or both. This formula works best if the family is involved with the therapy. Two or three sessions per week are all that is necessary.

Keep in mind; that if your child seems to respond well to the treatment but has not been able to solve their problems on their own, this may be a good option. Some children are hesitant when they first receive my answers to their questions. They may return to the same behavior to avoid being labeled "dumb." After a few weeks of therapy, they may begin working on the problems for themselves. You need to stick with it and not give up on your child.

Supporting your child through therapy is key. If your child is not willing to get help, no amount of counseling or tough love will convince them to seek treatment. Be understanding, but set limits and structure as needed. Be strong, don't give up, and you'll be amazed at your child's improvement.

All children need support, structure, and discipline. Your child will not get better without it. You may be overwhelmed by your child's behavior. Don't be afraid to ask for help. Talk to a school counselor or a teacher about your concerns. You will be happy you did. It is important to understand that it's normal for children to struggle with different emotions, especially intense negative ones such as anger and sadness. It's also normal for children to have intense negative emotions and dangerous impulsive behaviors when they experience life stressors such as bullying, abuse, neglect, etc. These problems can lead to serious problems over time.

Children must learn skills to control their emotions and healthily cope with life stressors. Many children need therapy to manage their problems. They need a therapist that specializes in DBT with children. DBT is a treatment for people of all ages, but it's most common for adolescents and young adults. Parents need to be involved with their child's treatment team to get the best results for the family.

It's essential that parents establish clear rules and guidelines, structure the home environment, and discipline their child appropriately when needed. Parents must provide emotional support to their children. It's important to remember that it takes a few weeks to see changes in your child. Give treatment time. Do not give up on your child. Support groups and family therapy can be valuable tools in the recovery process. They are best when used as part of a comprehensive treatment plan.

Children with DBT are happier, healthier, and more likely to succeed.

They are more likely to have solutions to their problems other than self-harm or suicide.

Remember, if you need help, talk to your doctor or a therapist. Treating children with DBT is a specialty. Ask your doctor for a referral if you need one. The most important thing for your child is to get them to treatment and work on the problems together.

Sometimes all a child needs are someone to listen. If the professionals involved with your child don't seem like they are listening, talk to another teacher, nurse, principal, neighbor, friend, or relative, or seek a second opinion.

There's nothing worse than a child not getting the help they need. It can be frustrating when your child is not progressing, but this doesn't mean it was all in vain. If you stick with treatment, patience, and support for your child, they will get better.

A few sessions of DBT with someone who specializes in DBT with children can provide you with a helping hand when it comes to dealing with your child's problems and behaving in ways that will help them reach their full potential.

Don't wait until your child is in crisis. Provide all the love, support, and structure you can. If your child has mild problems, it's best to start DBT early so there are no long-term issues or complications for your child. Keep all communication and documentation to a minimum. Ensure that all the professionals involved in the treatment are up-to-date on the treatment plan.

Ensure your child has a bedtime routine (especially important for children with impulsivity or self-mutilation issues) to help them get in order before bed. It's also important for children to have exposure to sunlight and get enough sleep.

Ensure your child gets seven to eight hours of sleep at night. If your child is having trouble sleeping, talk to the doctor about a solution. Some children have been prescribed Melatonin, but it can be habit-forming. Before using this method to help your child sleep, talk with the doctor first.

If you've tried everything else and nothing seems to work, then it may be time to consider DBT for your child (or you). This therapy has helped thousands of people and can help you and your child prevent behavioral problems in adulthood. It can help your child manage their emotions and problem-solving skills in a healthy way to improve their overall functioning.

If you have been through treatment with your child and failed at reaching your goals, you might find it difficult to get back on track. It's important to realize that the turmoil, stress, and depression you may feel in the process will be worth it if it leads to your child getting better. Unfortunately, no one magic pill will work for every child.

You may also feel lost and lonely as you try to figure out how to approach your child's treatment, who they are, and what they need after so many years without treatment. You may be at a loss regarding how to approach therapy with your child because they haven't gotten any worse, and there's no actual crisis.

It's also possible that you have tried other treatments which haven't worked. For some children, the symptoms of their depression might be so severe that they won't even seek help without encouragement from their parents. Remember that each child is different, so some people need much more treatment than others. Some may need more than one treatment or support to improve their behavior. DBT is an evidence-based treatment program for children under the age of 18.

You mustn't give up on your child. It's important to be patient and keep at it, even if your efforts seem futile. Many children will respond well to treatment with therapy. If it doesn't work, you can try another treatment or therapy. There are many different approaches to therapy; find the one that works best for you both as a team and as a family.

If you've tried all other methods and nothing seems to help, give DBT with someone who specializes in working with children with these issues a try — it might work for your child, too, and prevent many problems over the long term.

Set small goals and reach them. The most important thing is to concentrate on getting your child the needed help. You'll need a good family and friends support network who can hold you accountable for your children's treatment so that you don't slip up with your child's treatment. Don't be afraid to ask for professional help because this is essential in getting your child back on track. Working together as a team will make the process easier for everyone involved.

Make sure that the professionals involved with your child work together as a team and that there is coordination between all parties. This will ensure optimal outcomes and make it easier to treat your child.

Made in the USA
Monee, IL
26 November 2022

18479616R00079